A Parent's Guide to **Children's** Medicines

A Johns Hopkins Press Health Book

A Parent's Guide to **Children's** Medicines

Edward A. Bell, Pharm.D., BCPS

THE JOHNS HOPKINS UNIVERSITY PRESS • *Baltimore*

NOTE TO THE READER: This book describes medications as they are prescribed and given to children in general. It was not written about your child. The services of a competent professional should be obtained whenever medical or other specific advice is needed.

All efforts have been made to ensure the accuracy of the information contained in this book as of the date of publication. The author and the publisher expressly disclaim responsibility for any adverse outcomes arising from the use or application of the information contained herein.

© 2012 Edward A. Bell
All rights reserved. Published 2012
Printed in the United States of America on acid-free paper
9 8 7 6 5 4 3 2 1

The Johns Hopkins University Press
2715 North Charles Street
Baltimore, Maryland 21218-4363
www.press.jhu.edu

Library of Congress Cataloging-in-Publication Data

Bell, Edward A., 1959–
  A parent's guide to children's medicines / Edward A. Bell.
    p. cm. — (A Johns Hopkins Press health book)
  Includes bibliographical references and index.
   ISBN 978-1-4214-0623-7 (hdbk. : alk. paper) — ISBN 978-1-4214-0624-4 (pbk. :
  alk. paper) — ISBN 978-1-4214-0673-2 (electronic) — ISBN 1-4214-0623-3 (hdbk. :
  alk. paper) — ISBN 1-4214-0624-1 (pbk. : alk. paper) — ISBN 1-4214-0673-X (electronic)
  1. Pediatric pharmacology—Popular works. 2. Drugs—Popular works. I. Title.
   RJ560.B45 2012
   615.1083—dc23   2012000018

A catalog record for this book is available from the British Library.

Illustrations by Elizabeth Allen

*Special discounts are available for bulk purchases of this book. For more information,
please contact Special Sales at 410-516-6936 or specialsales@press.jhu.edu.*

The Johns Hopkins University Press uses environmentally friendly book materials,
including recycled text paper that is composed of at least 30 percent post-consumer
waste, whenever possible.

CONTENTS

Why I Wrote This Book

At some point, most parents have questions about how safe and useful a particular medication will be for their child. The medication may be available over the counter, like cough syrup, or it may be prescribed by a doctor, like an antibiotic. Parents want to know: Is the medication safe? Is it effective? Will it help my child? As a pediatric pharmacist for twenty-three years, I have listened carefully to these questions to identify the mother's or father's concerns. I hope I have given empathetic answers in reply—and my answers are always based on the latest scientific information.

The answers to the questions are usually, but not always, clear-cut. Many children's medicines are available today. These medications can effectively cure medical problems, prevent serious illnesses, or control chronic childhood problems such as asthma. Many medicines can greatly improve a child's life. All have the potential to cause side effects, however, and parents should understand these side effects.

Information from Web sites, magazine and newspaper articles, and advertising may be useful, but it may also be contradictory and misleading. It is easy for a parent to get confused. For example, many Internet sites inaccurately describe some medications as being dangerous to all children.

I decided to specialize in pediatric pharmacy because I enjoy working with children and talking with parents about their children's medications. As my own children grew up, my wife and I faced questions about whether they would benefit from using a medication. In this book I discuss many of the questions that parents have about medicines. I also address some of the concerns about children's medications that are raised in the newspapers and on television. I offer my professional opinion about using medications for various children's medical problems, and I discuss the science behind using medications, including results of scientific studies and the recommendations of professional medical organizations and the nation's pediatric medical experts.

It is my hope that this book will be able to help you, the parent, make informed decisions about what is best for your child when it comes to using any medicine.

*   *   *

This book would not have been possible without the support and advice from the following, whom I thank:

My wife and children, for their love and support.

The College of Pharmacy and Health Sciences of Drake University, for granting me sabbatical leave and the time to write this book.

The health care professionals of Blank Children's Hospital and Clinics.

The following individuals, for providing valuable advice and content review:

- Dr. Wendi Harris, pediatrician reviewer, Des Moines, Iowa
- Dr. Debra Bixler, pediatrician reviewer, Des Moines, Iowa
- Dr. Lynne G. Maxwell, Philadelphia, Pennsylvania
- Jolene McCoy, parent reviewer, Des Moines, Iowa
- Dr. Phil Brunell, Bethesda, Maryland.

The publishing staff of the Johns Hopkins University Press.

A Parent's Guide to **Children's** Medicines

CHAPTER 1

Should I Give Medicine to My Child?

"I don't like giving medicine to my child," many parents have told me, and I certainly understand their concerns. As a mother or father, you may be afraid of a medicine's side effects, or you may wonder if the medicine will help your child. In this chapter, I provide information you will want to consider. I also suggest questions you may ask your child's doctor and pharmacist when medicine has been recommended to treat your child's illness. This information can help you feel more comfortable that you are doing what is best for your child.

Some of the questions I discuss in this chapter are:

- What are the benefits of giving medicine to my child?
- What are the risks of giving medicine to my child?
- How do medicines work in a child, and how do they work differently in older children and adults?
- Are side effects of medicines similar in children and adults?
- Why are some medicines not appropriate for children?

What are the benefits and risks of giving medicine to my child?

Parents who don't like giving medicines to their child are probably concerned about the side effects of a medicine. Their concerns are understandable, especially if the child is an infant, because all medicines have the potential for side effects. Fortunately, the side effects of most medicines are not dangerous. The side effects of some medicines *may* be serious, however, so you should be familiar with the side effects that may occur with any medicine you give your child. When a medicine is given to an infant or child, it should have a benefit—to cure an illness or to make the child feel better. When thinking about whether to give medicine to your child, ask yourself: *What is the benefit and what is the risk of giving this medicine to my child?* The benefit of giving medicine to your child should be greater than the risk (the side effects).

What benefits do medicines have for my children?

Medicine can:

- cure an infection (for example, an ear infection),
- make your child feel better (for example, lower your child's fever),
- improve control of a chronic disease (for example, asthma), and
- prevent a serious illness (for example, measles).

Many medicines can be very effective and can greatly help your child.

Pediatricians and family doctors now have many effective medicines to choose from to treat a variety of childhood illnesses. Sometimes, however, a medicine may not help a child much. This might happen, for example, if a child has a serious disease that is difficult to treat. I've found that some parents "lose faith" in medicines when a specific medicine hasn't helped their child in the past.

It's important to understand the potential benefits and limitations—what might be called the *realistic benefits* of each medicine. The flu (influenza) vaccine, for instance, is effective at preventing a child from catching the flu. (*Effective* means that it works more than 50 percent of the time.) But the flu vaccine is better at preventing serious illness from the flu than it is at preventing flu. Children who have received a flu vaccine may still catch the flu and become ill, but they are less likely to be as sick as they would have been without the vaccine. In other words, the vaccine can prevent a child from becoming sicker, even though the vaccine may not prevent the child from catching the flu. When this happens, the flu vaccine did its job well, but parents may say, "The flu shot didn't help! My child still got the flu!" To avoid misunderstandings or disappointments, you should ask your doctor and pharmacist about the benefits of a medicine or vaccine when you are considering giving it to your child.

What side effects can a medicine have in a child?

All medicines can have side effects. The side effects of some medicines infrequently occur and are usually mild. Acetaminophen (Tylenol) is a good example. When acetaminophen is given correctly (the right amount for the child's age and weight, and at the right times), most children experience no side effects. Other medicines have many potential side effects, but the medicine can also be very helpful for the illness being treated. Prednisone is a good example. Prednisone is a strong anti-inflammatory steroid medicine that reduces swelling, and it can greatly help a child with breathing difficulties, such as asthma. But prednisone can cause difficulty sleeping and mood changes. Prednisone can also have some dangerous side effects, such as increased susceptibility to infection, but these occur only when prednisone is given in large doses (large amounts) for two weeks or longer. Parents might read about the dangers of some medicines without fully understanding how likely these side effects are.

Common side effects of many medicines are drowsiness, an upset stomach (including loose stools or diarrhea), or a headache. Often taking the medicine with food or lowering the dose can decrease the severity of these side effects. Ask your child's doctor and pharmacist what side effects may occur with a medicine that is recommended for your child, and what you may be able to do to lessen these effects. If a medicine helps your child and any side effects that occur are mild, then the benefit is greater than the risk.

What are the risks of not using medicine?

I've talked with some parents who are so afraid of side effects that they are hesitant to give certain medicines to their child—or will not give the medicines at all. For example, some parents of children with asthma are very concerned about the side effects of prednisone. Prednisone is effective in reducing breathing difficulties when a child with asthma is having an asthma attack (called an exacerbation). But, I mentioned above, prednisone can also cause hyperactive or moody behavior. When parents decide not to give their child prednisone because of their concerns about side effects, the child's breathing difficulties continue or even get worse, which can be dangerous, potentially even fatal, for a child with asthma.

Many parents have concerns about the risks of vaccines. The routinely recommended childhood vaccines, such as measles/mumps/rubella (MMR) and varicella (chicken pox), prevent serious infections and diseases. Some of these diseases do not occur often now, and it's easy for us to forget about them—they are "out of sight, out of mind." Yet it is still possible for a child to become sick with one of these infections, and a child who has not had the vaccine for that infection has a much higher risk of becoming sick, or even dying, from the disease. If you are worried about the side effects of a medicine or vaccination, discuss your concerns with your child's doctor and pharmacist. Ask what can be done to reduce the risk of side effects. Also ask about what risks are involved in *not* giving the medicine or vaccine to your child.

*

> The benefits of giving a medicine to your child should outweigh the risks of giving the medicine. Understand the benefits and side effects of a medicine before giving it to your child. Ask your child's doctor and pharmacist questions so you understand a medicine's benefits and side effects.

How does medicine work in my child's body?

Different types or classes of medicine work differently; they are said to have a specific action or mechanism for effectiveness. Some medicines attach to specific parts, called receptors, in the body. Other

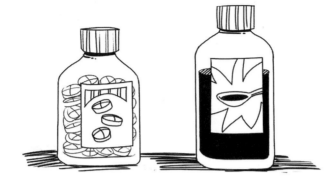

medicines change or decrease specific chemicals in the body. Ibuprofen (Motrin or Advil), for example, works to decrease specific chemicals that cause swelling and inflammation. Antibiotics work to kill harmful germs (bacteria). How a medicine works also explains the side effects it may cause. For example, albuterol (a common trade name is ProAir), a commonly used medicine for asthma that is taken by inhaler into the mouth, works by attaching to receptors in the lungs and other areas in the body. This medicine causes airways in the lungs to relax, or open up, allowing a person to breathe easier. However, because these receptors are also located in muscles, albuterol may cause some children to shake or have twitchy muscles, as a side effect.

Why do you need to know all of this? As a pharmacist, I believe that if you understand how a medicine works, you will better understand the potential benefits and side effects of the medicine. When I talk to children and their parents about their medicines, I try to help them understand how the medicine works, and how it will help them. I also let them know what side effects may occur. This information helps them make decisions and helps them cope if side effects occur.

How does medicine work differently in my child and in me?

Many medicines work differently in infants and children than they do in adults. These differences can result from how a medicine travels in a child's body, how it is metabolized (chemically changed) in a child's body, how it is eliminated from a child's body, and how it interacts with different parts of a child's body (table 1.1). An infant's or child's body differs in important ways from an adolescent's or an adult's body. The younger an infant or child is, the greater the differences in how medicines work. A well-known saying in pediatrics is that *children are not small adults*. For example, the percentage of water by body weight for an infant's body is greater than for an older child, adolescent, and adult. Many medicines travel to parts of the body where more water is located. Because an infant's body contains more water, the medicine will travel differently, and a different dose will have to be given for the medicine to work effectively. Scientists learn how medicines work differently in infants and children when they study or test medicines in infants and children. Many medicines are not studied in children, however.

What medicines should not be given to infants and children?

Some medicines may have different side effects in children than in adults. For example, aspirin should never be used to treat pain or fever in children younger than 18 years of age because it may cause Reye's syndrome. Reye's syndrome is a dangerous condition that affects the liver and brain. It is often fatal. Reye's syndrome usually occurs with a viral infection, such as chicken pox or influenza (the flu). Most people (90 percent or more) who contract Reye's syndrome have taken aspirin during the viral infection. Another medicine, tetracycline, which is an antibiotic, is not used in children under 9 years of age because it may stain developing teeth a grayish color.

Side effects for some other medicines occur less often in children than in adults. For example, a feared side effect of ibuprofen (Motrin, Advil) in adults, especially older adults, is a stomach ulcer, which can cause dangerous bleeding. While ibuprofen may also cause an ulcer in children, this very rarely occurs—certainly much less often than in adults. Older adults, however, must be careful using ibuprofen because of this side effect.

TABLE 1.1   How medicines work differently in infants, children, and adults

DIFFERENCE	INFANTS	CHILDREN	ADULTS
How medicine is absorbed into the body and bloodstream	• Greater percentage of water in skin compared to adults. • When swallowed, some medicines do not pass from the intestines into the bloodstream the same as in adults.	• When swallowed, some medicines do not pass from the intestines into the bloodstream the same as in adults.	
How medicine travels in the body	• With 70–75% of the body as water, some drugs travel more in the body than in adults.	• With 65–70% of the body as water, some drugs travel more in the body than in adults.	• With 55–60% of the body as water, some drugs travel less in the body than in children.
How medicine is changed in the body	• After being taken, some drugs are changed differently in the body as compared to adults.	• After being taken, some drugs are changed differently in the body as compared to adults.	

What can I do to reduce the potential for side effects when giving medicine to my child?

You can take several steps to avoid or minimize side effects. You can:

- Ask if the medicine is safe for infants or children. Ask if the medicine has been studied and tested in infants and children (for more on this topic, see below).

- If you decide to give the medicine, then give it as instructed by the doctor and the pharmacist. Don't give more than the recommended dose (more is not better for medicines), and don't give it more often. Some medicines cause side effects in children because they are not given correctly.

- Ask what side effects may occur and what to do if a side effect does occur.

- Ask if there is anything you can do to reduce the likelihood of side effects, such as giving the medicine with food.

*
All medicines can have side effects. Before giving a medicine to your child, ask what side effects may occur and what to do if they occur. Give the medicine to your child "as directed"—giving it exactly as it was explained to you will reduce the risk of side effects.

How are medicines tested in children?

Not all medicines *have* been studied in infants and children. In fact, only about 25 percent of medicines have been studied in infants and children; the other 75 percent are not officially "approved" for use in infants and children. What this means is that the Food and Drug Administration (FDA), the federal government's agency that regulates medication use and safety, has not officially stated that the drug has been adequately tested and studied in children. Fortunately, since the 1990s the Food and Drug Administration has put in place several important laws that are causing pharmaceutical companies to test more medicines in children. We will learn more about how specific medicines work in children over the coming years.

If a medicine is not "approved" for use in infants or children, it does not necessarily mean that the medicine is dangerous for children to take. When a medicine does not have FDA approval for use in infants or children, it usually means that the pharmaceutical company manufacturing the medicine has not tested it in children. Doctors can still prescribe a medicine for children even though it is not "approved" for children, and they frequently do.

The process of testing medicines in humans before they are commercially available for doctors to prescribe provides important information, such as how much of the medicine (what dose) works best and what side effects the medicine has. As I explained above, many medicines act differently in children than they do in adults. Thus, it is best to study medicines in infants and children, and not

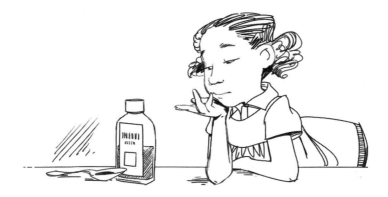

just in adults. You should not assume that medicines work the same in children and in adults. As you might imagine, it is more difficult and more expensive to study medicines in children. Many pharmaceutical companies do not test their medicines in children because they don't believe it will be profitable for them to do so. Some medicines are used every day in children, even though the pharmaceutical companies that make them have never tested them in children. Many of these medicines have been used in children for many years, or clinical researchers have studied them in children. Nevertheless, it is still best to use medicine that has been tested in children and shown to be safe in children. Ask your child's doctor and pharmacist if the medicine that has been recommended for your child has been tested in infants or children, and if it is FDA approved for use in children. If a medicine that your child's doctor recommends for your child is not FDA approved for children, ask if the medicine has been used in other children and if it is safe to use. Again, even though a medicine is not FDA approved for use in children, this does not necessarily mean that the medicine is dangerous. Discuss these issues with your child's doctor.

Case in point: Cough and cold medicine for children
A medicine illustrating the concern about testing medicines in children is over-the-counter cough and cold medicines. Pharmaceutical

companies that had long manufactured these medicines for infants and young children (younger than 4 years of age) stopped making them in 2008. Although these medicines were tested in adults, they were never tested in young children, so we didn't know if they were effective and safe in young children. In 2007 a group of physicians and a pharmacist asked the Food and Drug Administration to stop allowing over-the-counter cough and cold medicines to be sold for young children because there was no proof from medical studies that they were effective. In fact, there was evidence that they caused serious side effects. The FDA recommended not using over-the-counter cough and cold medicines in children under 2 years of age, and the pharmaceutical companies decided not to make them for children younger than 4 years of age. The FDA is now considering whether over-the-counter cough and cold medicines should be used for children 4 years of age and older.

*

Many medicines have not been studied in infants and children. Ask your child's doctor and pharmacist which medicines have been studied in infants and children and which medicine is best for your child.

CHAPTER 2

How Should I Give Medicine to My Child?

Let's assume that your child's doctor has recommended a specific medicine for your child. You have discussed how it can help your child, what side effects it may have, and whether it is safe to use in children. Next comes the art of giving the medicine to your child. This may not be as easy as it seems.

In this chapter, I answer these questions:

- If my child needs medicine, how can I get him or her to take it?
- What is the best way to measure liquid medicines accurately?
- What can I do to reduce my child's anxiety about, and pain from, an injection?

My son's doctor has prescribed a liquid medication.
Do all of them have a "medicine-y" taste?

One of the greatest frustrations you may face when giving medicine to your child is simply getting your son or daughter to take the medicine. Infants and young children do not understand that a medicine can help them feel better, so they may refuse to take it, especially if the medicine doesn't taste good. It's usually best to give a liquid medicine to infants and young children because they can't swallow tablets or capsules. For infants and young children, the taste of a liquid medicine is important. No one likes to swallow something that tastes bad!

Pharmaceutical companies flavor their liquid medicines to make them taste good. Some medicines are bitter, however, and their taste is difficult to mask, or cover up. Antibiotics are commonly used in children, and many are available as liquids. Researchers have done several "taste tests" of antibiotic medications, with the results published in medical journals. Liquid antibiotics that have been rated as tasting good are amoxicillin, Augmentin (amoxicillin-clavulanate), Omnicef (cefdinir), Cefzil (cefprozil), and Zithromax (azithromycin). Some liquid antibiotics have been rated as tasting bad (table 2.1). The same medicine can also differ in taste when made by different pharmaceutical companies. I've tried tasting many of these liquid antibiotics, and some of them taste pretty good, but unfortunately, not all of them do.

TABLE 2.1   Commonly used liquid antibiotics your child may not like because of taste

ANTIBIOTIC	FLAVOR
Biaxin (clarithromycin)	Fruit punch
Vantin (cefpodoxime)	Lemon crème
Ceftin (cefuroxime)	Tutti-frutti
Penicillin	Cherry
Clindamycin	Cherry

Most pediatricians and family doctors know which antibiotics taste better. Keep in mind that many factors besides taste determine the best antibiotic for your child, such as the type of infection and your child's age. Taste, while important, is only one factor. It's best not to insist that your child's doctor prescribe a specific antibiotic mainly because it tastes good. A liquid antibiotic that tastes good but is not the right one for your child's infection is not the best antibiotic for your child. Whenever your child needs any kind of liquid medicine, ask the doctor about the taste of the medicine that is prescribed.

Many children's over-the-counter medicines are available as liquids, and these, too, can have different tastes. Your pharmacist should be able to recommend one that tastes good. Keep in mind, of course, that taste can vary among children—what one child may like, another child may not like. I recall when my son was young and had a fever. We were out of acetaminophen (Tylenol), so I went to the pharmacy (of course it was late at night). I noticed that a generic form of infant's acetaminophen was much less expensive than the trade-name product, Tylenol, and I bought several boxes of the generic product. Well, my son must not have liked the taste because he wouldn't take the generic product. Back to the pharmacy I went to buy the trade-name product Tylenol. He liked this better and took it with much less complaining. I tried the tastes of both, and I agreed that the trade-name product Tylenol tasted better than the generic product.

A dosing syringe, despite its name, does not involve any needles. It is a measuring device and an oral delivery system all rolled into one. The adult can place the dosing syringe in the infant's or child's mouth and push down on the plunger to deliver the dose of medication gradually.

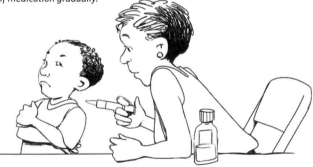

My son doesn't like the taste of a liquid medicine and will not take it. What can I do?

Many pharmacies are able to add flavorings to liquid medicines to improve their tastes. Ask your pharmacist if the pharmacy is able to flavor your child's liquid medicine. The flavorings most commonly used are made by the company FLAVORx. For a few extra dollars, the pharmacy can add flavorings to many medications, including liquid antibiotics. Commonly used flavors are bubblegum, chocolate, grape, wild cherry, and many others.

"Homemade" methods may also be used to improve the tastes of some medicines for older infants or young children (table 2.2). One method, which sounds quite good, is to give chocolate syrup as a "chaser" before or after a liquid medicine. A teaspoonful of chocolate syrup before and after the liquid medicine will "help the medicine go down." The syrup coats the tongue, helping to hide the taste of the medicine. Your son may also be willing to take the medicine when a treat follows. Other flavored syrups or liquids (for example, grape juice, butterscotch, or strawberry syrup) may also be used. Sugar-free chocolate syrups are also available.

TABLE 2.2   Homemade methods to improve a medicine's taste

Chocolate syrup	Give before or after medicine.
Juice	Use juice with a strong taste, such as grape juice.
Applesauce	Mix with the medicine.
Pudding	Mix with the medicine.
Popsicles	Give before or after medicine. Cold can hide a medicine's taste.

Another approach is to mix the liquid medicine with a small amount of chocolate syrup or other tasty liquid in a dosing syringe, spoon, or cup. Use a liquid with a strong taste, such as grape juice, which will help to mask the medicine's taste. Honey is another sweet liquid that can hide the taste of liquid medications. But a word of caution—use honey only if your child is older than 12 months because honey may contain certain germs that can be dangerous to young infants. You can also mix applesauce or pudding in with the medicine. Some parents give their older children popsicles before giving medicine. Not only does a cold popsicle taste good, but the cold temperature can numb taste buds on the tongue. Speaking of cold, keeping a liquid medicine in the refrigerator may make it taste better. Check with your pharmacist first, however, because some liquid medicines should not be stored in the refrigerator.

For infants taking infant formula, another method for administering medicines that don't taste good is to mix them in the bottle with the formula. But you should try the methods discussed above first, as the medicine may change the taste of your infant's formula, and he may not like the taste of the formula as much. Also, if your infant doesn't finish the whole bottle, he may not have gotten all of the medicine. Putting the bottle in the refrigerator for the next feeding may chemically change or weaken the medicine. So check with your pharmacist before doing this. If you do mix the medicine with infant formula, use a smaller amount of formula and give it to your infant when he is likely to be hungriest (perhaps the first feeding of the morning). If all goes well, he will drink the entire amount. Then you can give him the rest of his regular formula for that feeding.

For medicines only available as capsules or tablets, you can try to mix the capsule contents or crushed tablet with a strong tasting food (for example, jam or jelly) or a food your child will like (applesauce and pudding are often used). Some tablets should not be crushed, and some capsule contents should not be chewed (see below for more information about tablets and capsules). Be careful not to mix the medicine in too much of the food, as your child may not finish all of the food. Mix the medicine in just enough food to mask the taste but not too much for your child to finish. Also, do not combine the medicine with a tasty liquid or food and save it for later use, as the medicine may chemically change or weaken if left mixed with food for many hours. If you put medicine with a tasty food or liquid, do so just before giving it to your child.

Pharmacists may be able to take a medicine not typically available as a liquid and make it into a liquid at the pharmacy. To do this, they use pharmaceutical "recipes." Unfortunately, it's not as simple as crushing a tablet and mixing it with a good-tasting liquid. In a pharmaceutical recipe, the liquid made from tablets or capsules has been tested for being chemically stable; this means the drug does not lose its potency, or strength, when it is made into a liquid. If the medicine your child needs is not available as a liquid, ask your pharmacist if a recipe exists for making a liquid.

✻

> How a medicine tastes may be an important part of giving medicine to your child. Discuss a medicine's taste with your child's doctor. There are several methods available to improve a medicine's taste. Discuss these with your pharmacist.

What is the best way to measure out liquid medicine for my child?

Let's assume that the directions for your daughter's medicine tell you to give "one teaspoonful twice a day." How should you measure out "one teaspoonful?" Can you use a kitchen teaspoon? No! Why not? Kitchen teaspoons are not meant to be accurate measuring devices. Studies have shown that typical kitchen teaspoons may vary from 2 milliliters to 8 milliliters. A medical teaspoonful is 5 milliliters (ml). The American Academy of Pediatrics, the professional organization representing pediatricians, first cautioned parents not to use kitchen teaspoons for measuring liquid medicine in 1975.

Doctors commonly write prescriptions as "1 teaspoonful" or "1 tablespoonful." Some studies have shown that parents confuse teaspoonful with tablespoonful. One tablespoonful is the same as 3 teaspoonsful (15 ml)—so be careful.

Instead of a kitchen spoon, what device should you use to measure out your child's medicine? You can choose from several:

- dosing syringe
- dosing spoon
- dosing dropper (usually for smaller amounts, for infants)
- medicine cup

The best measuring device to use for one teaspoonful is a dosing syringe. Dosing syringes are often considered the best medicine-dosing device for infants and young children because they are easy to use and usually have markings in milliliters and teaspoonsful. Dosing syringes may also be placed into the child's mouth; that way, the adult can dispense the medicine slowly into the child's mouth.

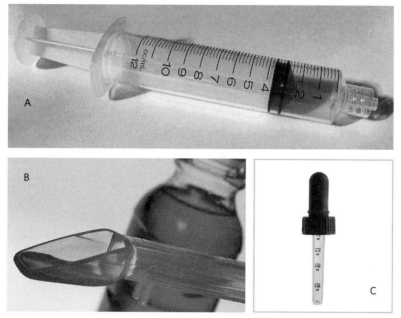

Three medicine dosing devices:
(A) a dosing syringe,
(B) a dosing spoon (definitely not a kitchen spoon), and
(C) a dosing dropper (for oral administration of a liquid medicine).

Infants have a natural suck instinct, and they often will suck the medicine out of the syringe.

Dosing syringes come in different sizes; smaller-sized ones are often the best device for measuring small amounts of liquid medicine (less than a teaspoonful, or 5 ml). Some dosing syringes come with a small cap; if you get one that has a cap, be careful with the cap (or throw the cap away) because it can be a choking hazard. Many doctor's offices have dosing syringes to give you, so ask for one. Many pharmacies will give parents dosing syringes if asked, or they will sell them inexpensively.

When giving medicine to your young child with a dosing syringe, point the syringe toward the side of your child's mouth and slowly push the medicine out. Do not point the syringe directly into the back of the mouth, as this may cause choking. Doctor's offices and pharmacies often have printed instruction sheets with diagrams of how to give oral medicines to infants and children. (See Appendix D for more information.) A dosing dropper, which can accurately measure small amounts of medicine, may be useful for infants. Alternately, you may use a dosing spoon, but it is easier to spill medicine from a dosing spoon. Dosing spoons are not as useful as droppers and syringes for young infants because the medicine has to be poured into the infant's mouth, which may easily lead to spilling.

Many liquid medicines purchased over the counter come with medicine cups. Research has found that some parents think they are supposed to give the entire full cup each time they give medicine to their child. Read the instructions and follow the age-appropriate dosing guide on the bottle or box of medicine. Use care with medicine cups because the numbers and lines on some of them are hard to see or read, making it difficult to measure liquid medicine accurately. It may be hard to measure out a small amount of medicine with a medicine cup, as thick liquid medicines are difficult to pour with a medicine cup into an infant's or child's mouth. Studies have shown that dosing syringes or droppers are more accurate than medicine cups. So use a dosing syringe, a dosing spoon, or a dosing dropper rather than a medicine cup.

If you need to give medicine to an infant or young child, you may find the Medibottle a useful dosing device. The Medibottle looks like a small formula bottle with a nipple, but it contains a dosing syringe built inside. The liquid medicine in the built-in dosing syringe mixes with formula or juice in the bottle, so that a child can swallow the medicine without difficulty, possibly not even knowing he was taking medicine. One study showed that Tylenol (acetaminophen) was easier to give to young infants (2 to 14 months) with a Medibottle than with a dosing syringe. A similar device is called ReliaDose. You can order either of these dosing devices from Internet sites, or your pharmacy may have them.

✳ Several devices can be used to give liquid medicine to your infant or young child. A dosing syringe is accurate and easy to use. Do not use kitchen teaspoons or tablespoons to give liquid medicine.

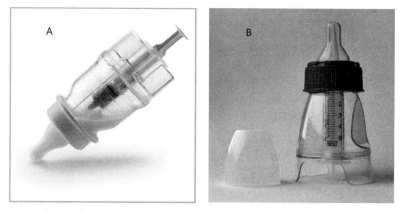

(A) Medibottle (courtesy of the Medicine Bottle Company) and
(B) ReliaDose (courtesy of Blaine Pharmaceuticals, Inc.; photo by Shelley Rees).

What should I do if my daughter vomits right after I give her medicine?

This is a common question. The answer depends on the specific medicine given and how much time passed between when she took the medicine and when she vomited. Parents are often told that if it has been less than one hour since giving the medicine, then they should give another dose of the medicine. This may not be true for all medicines, however. Liquid medicines may be absorbed into the bloodstream faster than tablets or capsules. Most liquid medicines are absorbed into the bloodstream in less than one hour. If a child is given a liquid medicine and vomits 45 minutes later, giving another dose of the medicine probably isn't necessary. If the medicine was a tablet or capsule, it can be helpful—although unpleasant—to look at your child's vomit. If you see large pieces of the tablet or capsule, then most of it probably wasn't absorbed, so you can give another tablet or capsule.

The specific type of medicine is important to consider. Some medicines may have dangerous side effects if too much of the medicine is given. Other medicines, such as liquid antibiotics, are not as dangerous when more is given. Call your doctor or pharmacist if your child vomits soon after being given medicine, and ask if you should give more medicine.

My son's doctor prescribed a medicine that comes only as a tablet. If my son can't swallow the tablet, may I split or crush it?

Many—but not all—medicines that come as tablets and capsules may be split, crushed, or opened up and given to a child. However, some tablet medicines have a special coating that should not be broken before they are swallowed. Some capsules may be opened and the contents mixed with soft food, such as applesauce. However, the tiny beads or contents of the capsule often should not be chewed. Some tablets can be split or cut in half, which may help if your child can swallow a smaller tablet piece. Tablets with a grooved line in the middle (called "scored" tablets) are easier to cut or split. There are many devices you can buy to split or crush a tablet easily. Some can both cut and crush tablets, and they can also store several tablets. For just a few dollars you can buy tablet splitters and crushers at many pharmacies and from various Internet sites. Always check with your pharmacist before breaking or crushing tablets or opening capsules.

Many parents ask me when their children should be able to swallow their medicine. The answer is that it varies a lot. Some parents of young children, 3 or 4 years old, have told me that their child can swallow tablets. I know of other parents whose child is 10 or 11 years old, or even older, and cannot swallow a tablet. Even some adolescents and adults find it hard to swallow tablets or capsules whole. Medical textbooks state that children should be able to swallow tablets and capsules at about age 6 or 7 years.

There are devices you can buy to help your child learn how to swallow a tablet or capsule. One device, called Oralflo, is similar to a small cup with a spout (like a young child's sippy cup). Inside the spout is an area that holds a tablet. When the child drinks from the cup, the tablet slides into the child's mouth with the liquid, making it easier for the child to swallow the tablet. I have seen similar looking "swallowing" cups with spouts in doctor's offices that pharmaceutical companies provide as giveaways for parents. Ask at your child's doctor's office if they have these cups. Many pharmacies sell them as well.

My son is afraid of getting a shot when I take him to our pediatrician. What can I do?

"Getting a shot" is the greatest fear children have when in a doctor's office. Many of the routinely recommended vaccines are given early in childhood, and children remember the anxiety and discomfort of receiving these vaccines. Often the anxiety leading up to getting a shot is worse for the child—and the parent—than the actual discomfort of the needle poke. A needle poke for taking blood, or putting in an intravenous (IV) line, may be even more painful to a child. There are children who require two or three adults to hold them down to get a shot. Children often begin to get upset at home, well before the doctor's appointment, anticipating getting a shot. What can you do to calm your child?

Several techniques can help comfort your infant or child during needle pokes or vaccine shots. Medical studies have evaluated the parental behavior that is most likely to reduce a child's discomfort and anxiety. One medical study found that 53 percent of a change in a child's distress during administration of a vaccine was due to the mother's behavior. In other words, the mother's behavior can be helpful, or not helpful, when a child is upset about getting a shot. Some parental behaviors that have been shown to be helpful include humor and distraction (such as telling stories, reading to the child, showing a movie, using party blowers, or blowing bubbles). Techniques such as being empathetic, apologizing, or giving control to your child have been shown to *increase* a child's distress during shots or other painful procedures. Several studies have tested whether reassurance is helpful to a child, and although it did help some children, many children had more distress from reassurance. Distraction may be one of the best techniques a parent can use. For infants younger than 6 months, giving the infant sugar water (sucrose) may help reduce pain from shots and other painful procedures. One packet of sugar mixed with 10 ml (2 teaspoonsful) of water may be placed into your infant's mouth with a medicine syringe or placed onto a pacifier. Using sugar water and a pacifier, along with parental contact (holding or caressing your infant), may be more helpful for a young infant. Studies have shown that giving sugar water may still be helpful, but likely will not work as well, when infants are 4 to 6 months of age or older. Use of a pacifier alone has also been shown to help relieve pain in young infants.

Several medicines are available (by prescription and over the counter) that may reduce or even eliminate the pain from a needle poke. These numbing medicines are available as creams and ointments, or as a patch that may be placed on your child's skin (where the needle is likely to be given) at home. They begin to work in about 20 to 60 minutes, and they numb the skin by the time the needle poke is given in the doctor's office. I frequently recommend these numbing creams to parents. Their names are EMLA, LMX-4, and Synera. You can buy LMX-4 without a prescription, although it is rather expensive (about $40 to $50). Some doctor's offices may have other numbing medicines or cooling sprays that they use. Synera and LMX-4 should be applied to a child's skin at least 20 or 30 minutes before the needle poke, and EMLA should be applied at least 60 minutes before the needle poke.

Because these medicines have to be placed onto your child's skin well before the needle poke, some planning is necessary. It may be best to place them on your child at home, as they won't start working for 30 to 60 minutes. Because the injection spot on your child can vary (due to your child's age, or where a "good" vein can be found), ask your doctor's office staff for their recommendation on where to place the numbing medicine. Sometimes it is best to place the medicine on several different sites on your child, just in case a "good

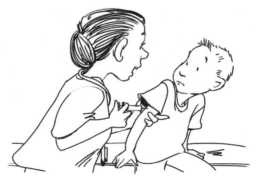

No one likes to get a shot, but there are techniques that may ease a child's anxiety and pain.

vein" can't be found on the first try. Common spots to place these medicines include the antecubital area (inside part of the arm, across from the elbow) or the back of the hand. It is important to follow the directions for these medicines carefully because each medicine should be applied differently.

*

Getting a shot is the biggest fear children have when in a doctor's office. Numbing medicines used on your child's skin may lessen the pain of a needle poke. Ask your doctor or pharmacist about these medicines. You can also help by using certain behaviors with your child.

CHAPTER 3

How Do I Use Medicines for Fever?

In this chapter I discuss one of the most common reasons parents call or visit their child's doctor: fever. When your child has a fever, you may wonder:

- How high can my child's fever go?
- Is a high fever dangerous?
- What medication is best for treating my child's fever?
- How much medication should I give? Am I giving too much medication?

Fever itself is not a disease—it is a symptom of some type of problem, or insult, to the body. Fever usually results from an infection. A fever does not always mean that a serious illness is present. However, a fever may occur because of some dangerous infections, so it is important to watch your child closely when he or she has a fever and to speak frequently with your child's doctor. A fever can make your child uncomfortable, which is usually the most important reason to treat it. It is important to contact your child's doctor or nurses when your child has a fever so they can determine how serious the illness may be and whether you should bring your child to the doctor's office or to a hospital emergency room.

Children have high fevers from illnesses more commonly than adults do, and children usually don't seem as uncomfortable as adults do with higher fevers. In other words, children usually tolerate higher fevers much better than we adults do.

What temperature do doctors consider to be a fever?

A fever is an increase in body temperature greater than normal because of a problem with the body, which is usually due to an infection. What temperature do doctors consider to be a fever? A body temperature of 100.4°F (38°C) or higher usually indicates a fever. Young infants (about 3 months of age and younger) may not be able to develop as high a fever as older infants or children. So some doctors may tell parents that even a fever less than 100.4°F in young infants can still mean that a serious infection is present.

Since 98.6°F is considered normal body temperature, you may wonder, "Isn't a temperature of 99°F a fever?" It's normal for a child's body temperature to vary over the course of a day. A child's body temperature can change due to the temperature of the room or outside air, the activity of the child, or the time of day. For example, if your child is playing outside on a warm summer day, he or she may have a body temperature greater than 98.6°F, but it's unlikely that means he or she has a fever or is sick.

What causes a fever and what happens when a fever is present?

Although many factors can cause a fever, a fever most commonly results from an infection of some type. The area of the brain that controls body temperature is called the hypothalamus. Think of the hypothalamus as the body's thermostat. Viruses or bacteria (germs) usually cause infection in infants and children, and these infections cause the immune system (the part of our body that helps to protect us) to make certain chemicals that increase the body's temperature. Just like when you turn up the thermostat in a room, it causes the temperature to rise. Again, a fever is not a disease; it is a symptom of some type of problem, which, in children, usually is an infection. Many parents believe that a fever will continue to rise unless it is treated, but this is not true. When your child has a fever, his or her temperature will rise but only to the new "set point" in the hypo-thalamus. Adjusting a room's thermostat from 75°F (comfortable) to 83°F (feels warm) will cause the air temperature to rise to 83°F but no further. The hypothalamus works the same way.

When your child has a fever, she may feel cold and shiver, or she may want to be under a blanket. This is because her body is trying to make more heat as the "thermostat" is turned up. Her heart rate and breathing rate can increase, and she may not feel like eating or drinking. If you give a medication such as Tylenol (acetaminophen), or if the immune system destroys the bacterial or viral infection, the "set point" is then lowered, but the fever may remain high for a time. Your child feels warm and her blood vessels dilate (become wider) to release heat. This may cause the skin to look red or flushed and the child to sweat.

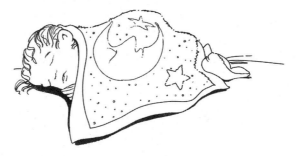

My neighbor is a nurse, and she told me that a fever can actually be good for my child. Is this true?

For most children, a fever is not dangerous. What's most important to consider is "What is causing my child's fever?" or "Is the cause of my child's fever dangerous?" This is what your child's doctor is thinking about—it's *what's causing the fever*, not the fever itself, that matters. For example, a fever from a cold is different from a fever from meningitis (a dangerous infection of the brain), as meningitis can quickly kill a child. Fortunately, viruses that are not dangerous, such as the viruses that cause colds, cause most fevers in children.

A fever may be dangerous if it leads to severe dehydration. Sweat-ing and loss of appetite from fever may cause your child to drink less and lose more body fluid. When your child drinks and eats less, or is vomiting, it is easy for him to become dehydrated. And it can be dangerous for a child to become too dehydrated. Children with fever also lose body fluid from sweating, which also can cause dehydration.

Again, a fever by itself in *most children* is not usually dangerous. But in some children, including children with certain congenital (born with) heart problems, lung diseases, metabolic diseases, or other serious diseases, a fever may be more dangerous. In children with diseases of the immune system, infections that may cause a fever may be especially dangerous. If your child has one of these medical problems, it is more important to be in close contact with your child's doctor.

Some experts believe that a fever may actually be good for your child. How can this be? Studies with animals have shown that when a fever is present, the immune system is better able to kill the germs causing the fever. Some studies with animals also show that germs do not reproduce as well in the body when the body temperature is higher. Animals with an infection and fever live longer compared to animals with an infection when the fever is lowered with medication. This may be one way that Mother Nature protects us from the dangers of infections.

---

*

A fever is usually not dangerous, and a fever even may be good for your child. What is causing the fever is what's important. An infant or child with a fever can easily become dehydrated.

When you call your child's doctor, he or she will probably ask you questions about how ill your child is, such as:

- "How is your child's activity level? Is he behaving normally?"
- "Is he alert?"
- "Is he drinking or eating?"
- "Does he respond to you?"

If your child has a fever but otherwise seems relatively normal, then your child's doctor probably will allow your child to stay at home and be treated with fever medication. However, if your child seems "out of it" or is not alert, then the doctor will probably ask you to bring him or her to the doctor's office or a hospital emergency room. Younger infants (younger than about 3 to 6 months of age) can become sicker more quickly than older infants, so your doctor may want to see or examine younger infants. A fever, even a low fever, in a young infant can be a sign of a dangerous infection. Although it is important to speak frequently with your child's doctor when your child has a fever, it is even more important when the child is a young infant.

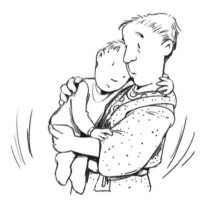

Do I have "fever phobia"?

It is understandable and normal to be concerned if your child has a fever. Some parents become overly concerned, however, and may believe that a fever is more dangerous than it actually is. This can cause the parent to give too much medicine. In the 1980s a pediatrician named Dr. Barton Schmitt from the University of Colorado noticed that his patients' parents seemed overly worried about fever in their children. He surveyed these parents in his clinic and found that many of them had fears about fever that were not medically true. Dr. Schmitt called these fears "fever phobia." For example, many parents believed that a high fever could cause brain damage, or that the exact number of the temperature is important, or that fevers over 104°F are dangerous.

In 2001, other doctors surveyed parents with similar questions about fever and found that these parents also had "fever phobia." For example, 85 percent of parents said that they would wake their child up at night to give him or her medicine for fever, and 44 percent of parents—almost half—gave the fever medicine ibuprofen (Motrin, Advil) too often.

Many of these parents' fears are not medically true for fevers caused by infection and other common medical problems. For example, a body temperature as high as 107.6°F has not been shown to cause brain damage. When a very high temperature (greater than 106°F to 107°F) occurs in a child, which happens rarely, a medical condition called hyperthermia is more likely to be the cause. Fevers from infection very rarely cause such high temperatures. When your child has a fever, try not to focus on the temperature number itself but instead on what other symptoms she has. Is she drinking enough fluid? Is she alert and acting normal? And, of course, stay in contact with your child's doctor.

I recall when my son was about 5 years old and wasn't feeling well. His cheeks were quite red, and when I touched his face, he felt like a hot iron! His temperature was 105°F! Even with this high temperature, he was sitting up and watching cartoons on television, and he could answer questions I asked him. He felt better in a few days.

What is the best way to measure my child's temperature?

How we take a child's temperature has changed a lot over the years. Mercury thermometers, which for many years were the most common way of measuring temperature, should no longer be used. The American Academy of Pediatrics recommends not keeping mercury thermometers in the home. This is because mercury can be dangerous if the thermometer breaks. There are several types of thermometers you can buy. The main factor determining which type to use for your child is his or her age (table 3.1).

The main types of thermometers are digital probe, tympanic

TABLE 3.1   Types of thermometers to measure temperature in infants and children

TYPE OF THERMOMETER	COMMENTS
Digital probe	Can be used rectally, orally, or under arm (axillary).
Tympanic (ear)	Used in the ear. Many doctor's offices use this type of thermometer.
Temporal artery (infrared)	Measures temperature on skin over the temporal artery (forehead area).
Pacifier thermometers	Can be difficult to keep in place in an infant's mouth.
Temperature strips	May not be accurate. Don't use.

(ear), and temporal artery (infrared). Many people use digital probe thermometers because they are usually accurate and usually inexpensive. Digital probe thermometers can be used to take rectal, oral, or axillary (under arm) temperatures. For young infants (under 3 months of age), temperature should be taken only rectally. Infants age 3 to 36 months can have their temperature taken rectally or under the arm. Temperature may be measured orally for children when they are about 4 years of age.

You can also buy a pacifier thermometer, for use in infants. A pacifier thermometer may seem convenient, but it needs to stay in place in the infant's mouth for several minutes to be accurate, and achieving this may be difficult. Temperature strips that are placed on the skin are also available, but they are not accurate and should not be used. Whatever type of thermometer you use, it is important to follow the directions for that specific thermometer carefully, as the various types of thermometers are used differently.

Many doctors consider rectal temperature to be the most accurate measure of body temperature, but taking a temperature rectally may be difficult or uncomfortable for your child for obvious reasons. Other doctors consider tympanic temperature measurement to be the most accurate because the temperature of the blood near the tympanic membranes (ear drums) is very similar to the temperature of the blood near the hypothalamus (the body's thermostat). Tympanic thermometers are commonly used in many doctor's offices.

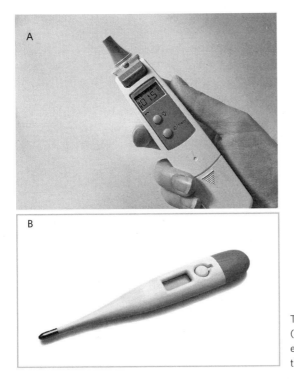

Two thermometers:
(A) tympanic (for use in the ear) and (B) a digital probe thermometer.

Tympanic thermometers are accurate, though a buildup of earwax in a child's ear may make them less accurate, and they need to be placed into the ear just right to work correctly. When using a tympanic thermometer, be sure to follow the instructions carefully.

When taking your child's temperature, keep in mind that temperature may vary by how the temperature is taken. A rectal temperature is usually about 1°F higher than an oral temperature, and an oral temperature is usually about 1° or 2°F higher than an axillary temperature. So, a child with a temperature of 99°F taken under the arm has an oral temperature of 100° to 101°F.

Here's another important point to keep in mind: the old-fashioned method of touching your child's forehead or face to see if he or she "has a temperature" is not accurate, and several studies have shown this. I remember when my mother used to check me for fevers this way. If your child feels warm and seems uncomfortable, use a thermometer to take his or her temperature accurately.

Should I give medicine to my child to try to lower his temperature to 98.6°F?

It's easy to understand a parent wanting to lower his or her child's temperature to 98.6°F when the child has a fever. However, it is not usually necessary to do so. Trying to lower your child's temperature to 98.6°F actually may do more harm than good, as you may give too much medicine without realizing it. Fever medicines generally will lower a child's temperature by about 2 to 3°F at most. Say your child has a fever of 103°F; you give fever medicine, and the temperature goes down to about 100°F. You may then want to give more fever medicine to lower the temperature even more, and you give too much medicine. A child whose temperature is lowered from 103°F to 100°F will likely feel more comfortable, and generally there is no need to try to lower the temperature further. What is most important is making your child comfortable and having him or her feel better.

If your child has other medical problems that may make fever more dangerous, lowering your child's temperature to 98.6°F, or close to it, may be more important. You should speak with your child's doctor about this.

As I discussed earlier in this chapter, a fever may cause your child's heart rate and breathing rate to increase, and he or she may not feel like eating or drinking, which can easily cause your child to become dehydrated. When your child begins to feel better, he or she will probably want to drink or eat more. Also, infants and children are more likely to sleep better when their fever is down and they are more comfortable.

Besides medicine, there are other ways you can help your child feel more comfortable during a fever. Children with a fever sweat more and often don't feel like drinking or eating, so it's important to encourage your child to drink fluids to prevent dehydration. If your child is already dehydrated, your doctor may want you to give him or her a special drink called oral rehydration solution (for example, Pedialyte). You can buy oral rehydration solution in a pharmacy and in many grocery stores without a prescription, and it comes in different flavors (for more about oral rehydration solutions, see chapter 6).

If your child is warm and uncomfortable, reduce the number of clothing layers he has on. If your child has a higher fever, you may think it would be a good idea to give him a cool bath. However, a cool bath does not lower a fever, and it may actually cause him to shiver and be more uncomfortable. Don't ever use cool water in a bath, and never add rubbing alcohol to the bathwater in an attempt to provide cooling action. Your child's skin may absorb the alcohol, causing potentially dangerous side effects.

> It is more important to give medicine to your child to make him or her feel more comfortable than to try to lower his or her temperature to normal. Your child's temperature does not have to be lowered to 98.6°F for him or her to feel better.

Can I use aspirin to treat my child's fever?

No! Aspirin should never be used to treat a fever in an infant, child, or even an adolescent younger than 18 years. Although aspirin can lower a fever, and it can be used in adults to lower fever, using aspirin in children to lower fever has been associated with a potentially fatal medical condition called Reye's syndrome. Some medication products may contain aspirin or salicylates (the chemical class of aspirin). Check with your pharmacist if you are not sure if a medication product you have contains aspirin (also known as acetylsalicylic acid).

I have both acetaminophen (Tylenol) and ibuprofen (Motrin, Advil) at home. Which one should I use for my child's fever? Which one is better?

Acetaminophen (the most common trade name is Tylenol) and ibuprofen (the most common trade names are Motrin and Advil) are the anti-fever medicines you can use to treat fever in your child or infant. Many parents wonder which one to buy. There are some differences between them, and which one to use depends on several factors. One factor is the age of your child. Acetaminophen can be used at any age, even at day 1 of life. However, if you have a young infant (younger than about 3 to 6 months) who has a fever, speak with your doctor before you give him or her acetaminophen. As explained earlier in this chapter, younger infants may have more serious infections and may need to be examined by a doctor.

Ibuprofen should not be given to an infant under 6 months of age. This is not because of any special problems that ibuprofen causes or dangers that it poses when given to younger infants. It is only because ibuprofen has been tested in infants 6 months of age and older, and the Food and Drug Administration has given its approval to use ibuprofen in infants over age 6 months. Ibuprofen may also not be best for your child if he or she has kidney disease, or if your child is dehydrated or has certain medical problems in the digestive tract, such as an ulcer.

Many scientific studies comparing acetaminophen and ibuprofen in infants and children have been published in medical journals. Most studies have found the two drugs to be equally effective, although a few studies concluded that ibuprofen was more effective than acetaminophen in reducing fever. These studies generally evaluated how much or how quickly the medicine helped lower temperature in children with fever. They did not usually measure which drug made children feel more comfortable. Some doctors may instruct parents to use ibuprofen for higher fevers, implying that it is more effective than acetaminophen. I consider acetaminophen and ibuprofen to be equally effective—they both work well to lower a child's fever.

As every child is different, it is possible that your child may do better when given acetaminophen, or it may be that ibuprofen works better for him or her. Most pediatric textbooks state that acetaminophen is the "drug of choice" for treating fever in infants and children. This is because the medical community (doctors, pharmacists, and nurses) has many years of experience using acetaminophen, and we know that it works well and is safe to use. But ibuprofen can be used before acetaminophen in older infants. If your child is 6 months of age or older, you can use either acetaminophen or ibuprofen.

When using acetaminophen or ibuprofen, it is important to have reasonable expectations about how much either medication will lower your child's fever. Don't expect either medicine to lower your child's temperature to 98.6°F. Parents who expect medication to lower a fever to 98.6°F may end up giving too much medication. So, if your child has a temperature of 104°F, acetaminophen or ibuprofen will likely lower his or her temperature to about 101°F. As noted above, acetaminophen and ibuprofen will usually lower a child's temperature about 2 or 3°F when a fever is present. Again, the goal of treating fever is making your child more comfortable, not necessarily lowering his or her temperature to 98.6°F.

> Both acetaminophen and ibuprofen are effective fever medicines. These medicines may not lower your child's temperature to 98.6°F. The goal of giving fever medicine to your child is to make him or her more comfortable, not to lower temperature to 98.6°F.

How much acetaminophen or ibuprofen should I give my child?

Knowing how much acetaminophen or ibuprofen to give your child—this is called the *dose*—is important. It's easy to give either too little or too much medicine. Parents may not be sure how much acetaminophen or ibuprofen to give, especially to a young infant. The child may develop fever late at night or on a weekend, and parents may not want to call their child's doctor. Several medical studies have shown that parents commonly do not give a large enough dose of a fever medicine to their child because they are not sure how much to give. The problem with not giving a large enough dose of acetaminophen or ibuprofen to your child is that it will probably not lower his or her fever. This may cause you either to give more and more of the medicine or to bring your child to a hospital emergency room, which may not be necessary.

The best way to determine how much acetaminophen or ibuprofen your child should have is to use his or her weight as a guide. The normal dose for acetaminophen is 10 to 15 milligrams (mg) per kilogram of body weight. One kilogram is equal to 2.2 pounds. Put another way, give 4.5 to 6.5 mg of acetaminophen per pound of body weight. Usually we health care workers give medications to children using kilograms as the measure of body weight because the normal dosing numbers are easier to remember (i.e., 10–15 instead of 4.5–6.5). You may give acetaminophen every 4 to 6 hours, but do not give more than 5 doses in a 24-hour period. The amount of ibuprofen to give your child is 5 to 10 mg per kilogram (2.5–4.5 mg per pound), every 6 to 8 hours.

Note that ibuprofen lasts somewhat longer than acetaminophen—up to 8 hours, as compared to 6 hours for acetaminophen. This can be an important difference, especially if your child has trouble taking medicines. Giving ibuprofen at bedtime may allow your child to sleep better if the fever is lowered for a longer time. If your child sleeps better, you sleep better.

Acetaminophen and ibuprofen can also be dosed by your child's age, and this is commonly done. However, this method is not as accurate as dosing by weight because children of the same age can have very different body weights. Acetaminophen and ibuprofen products list on the bottle and packaging how much medicine to give by age and a range of weight. For example, for a 2- to 3-year-old child with a weight between 24 and 35 pounds, the packaging for an acetaminophen children's liquid would recommend a dose of 160 mg of medicine. If you are not sure how much medicine to give, call a local pharmacy and ask a pharmacist. Many pharmacies are open 24 hours. You should tell them your child's age, weight, and what medicine product you want to use. Of course, you may also call your doctor's office for help.

Here are two other important points about how much fever medicine to give your child. First, children younger than 2 years can have rapid increases of weight over several months. This means that a dose of acetaminophen or ibuprofen that was accurate for your child's weight several months ago may now be too low. I've spoken with many parents who were not giving enough fever medicine to their child because they were giving an amount that was accurate for their child's weight from a few months earlier. If it has been several months since you last gave fever medicine to your child, the amount of medicine to give now is probably higher than the last time you gave it. Second, doses of fever medicine for older children or adolescents are likely to be the same as for an adult. When a child's dose of fever medicine, based on his or her weight, is larger than a usual adult dose, you should *give the adult dose,* not the larger dose.

Should I alternate giving acetaminophen and ibuprofen to my child? Is it better to give both acetaminophen and ibuprofen together?

Some parents alternate giving doses of acetaminophen and ibuprofen to their child. For example, they give acetaminophen, then 4 hours later give ibuprofen, and then repeat this. This allows parents to give the medicine more frequently. Some doctors recommend this dosing. Until several years ago, there were no medical studies to show that this method was better than giving just one medicine alone. Since then, a few medical studies testing alternating acetaminophen and ibuprofen have shown that alternating the two medicines lowered fever a little bit more (by about 1°F) than just giving one medicine alone. Many other experts, however, believe that alternating fever medicines may cause more side effects. It is possible that acetaminophen and ibuprofen may interact in the body when used together and cause more side effects. Also, alternating acetaminophen and ibuprofen can be confusing, and some studies have shown that parents may accidentally give too much fever medicine this way.

I don't believe that it is necessary to alternate acetaminophen and ibuprofen for most children. Many experts believe, as do I, that parents should give only one fever medicine to their child. I believe alternating acetaminophen and ibuprofen may be confusing and may unnecessarily cause a mistake. What about giving acetaminophen and ibuprofen together at the same time? One study was done to find out whether giving both medicines was better than giving each medicine alone. The combination of both medicines was found to be no better at treating a child's fever than giving acetaminophen or ibuprofen alone. When your child has a fever, use either acetaminophen or ibuprofen alone and be sure to give the right amount, as explained above.

What are the "take home" points about fever medicines?

First, *fever by itself is not necessarily bad; it may in fact be good for* your child. Don't have "fever phobia." However, *higher fevers may be a sign of a dangerous infection* and deserve a phone call to your pediatrician or family doctor. (Many pediatricians consider a high fever to be 104°F or greater.)

Second, if you give acetaminophen or ibuprofen, be sure to *give an accurate amount—based on your child's weight.* Ask your pharmacist or doctor for help in determining an accurate amount of medicine.

Third, *the goal of giving fever medicine is to make your child more comfortable,* not to lower his or her temperature to 98.6°F. The goal of treating fever is to improve your child's comfort and to have him or her drink fluids and feel better. It is not necessary to return a temperature to normal to achieve this.

When I am in the pharmacy to buy fever medicine, it is confusing because there are so many different fever medicines for children. Which one should I buy for my child?

There are many different types, or dosage forms, of acetaminophen or ibuprofen you can buy for your child (table 3.2). (A "dosage form" means what form the medicine is in, such as liquid, chewable tablet, or a swallowable tablet.) Probably the most important factor in deciding which product is best for your child is his or her age. The products differ by how much medicine they contain (the concentration). These different products are meant to be used for different ages. You can buy ibuprofen as a more concentrated liquid, described on the medicine package as "infants' suspension." These infant products are more concentrated than the children's liquid products; that is to say, the liquid contains more milligrams of the drug per volume of liquid. The infants' suspension is more concentrated so that a parent does not have to give a lot of liquid medicine to an infant; infants are more likely to choke on a large volume of liquid because their mouths are smaller. Acetaminophen is available as infants' liquid and children's liquid products. However, in 2011 the Food and Drug Administration recommended that the concentration of infant acetaminophen products be changed to the same concentration as the children's product. This was done to try to prevent parents from mistakenly giving too much acetaminophen. Before this, the infants' liquid product was three times as concentrated as the children's liquid. Most manufacturers of infant acetaminophen products, but perhaps not all, have changed the concentration to the same as the children's product. You may still have some of the older infants' liquid acetaminophen products in your home. The concern was that parents might accidentally give their child the more concentrated infants' product when the dose (amount of liquid) they determined was based on the amount of medicine in the children's product, which is less concentrated (contains less medicine).

For ibuprofen (Motrin, Advil), the infants' product contains 50 mg in 1.25 ml, which is the equivalent of 40 mg in 1 ml. The children's ibuprofen product contains 100 mg per 5 ml, the equivalent of 20 mg in 1 ml. So, the infants' product is twice as concentrated as the children's liquid product, again so a smaller volume of liquid can be given to an infant to prevent choking.

There is no specified age when parents should begin using the children's liquid products instead of the infants' liquid products. Generally, you can consider using the children's liquid products when your child is about 2 years old. What is most important, however, is that you be aware which product you are using and that you be sure the amount of liquid medicine you give is accurate—that the dose contains the right amount of medicine for your child's weight. One medical survey of parents' knowledge of fever medicines found that many parents assumed that children's liquid was more concentrated than infants' liquid—they thought that because children were bigger, children's liquids should have more medicine in them. This shows how confusing using the different fever medicines can be, and how easy it can be to make a mistake by giving your child too little or too much medicine.

You can buy acetaminophen as chewable or melt-away tablets (which melt or dissolve on the tongue) and ibuprofen as chewable tablets. These easy-to-use tablets can be useful for older children who don't want to take liquid medicine. However, these chewable and melt-away tablets also come in different amounts, so pay attention to how much medicine (how many milligrams) is in these products when you buy and use them. Two strengths are available

TABLE 3.2 Fever medicine for infants and children

DRUG	AMOUNT TO GIVE	HOW OFTEN TO GIVE	DIFFERENT PRODUCTS AVAILABLE	COMMENTS
Acetaminophen • Tylenol • generic	• Give amount by weight—this is more accurate than by age. • 10–15 mg per kilogram, or 4.5–6.5 mg per pound of body weight.	• Every 4–6 hours; no more than 5 doses in 24 hours.	• Infants' liquid and children's suspension (same concentration—160 mg per 5 ml 1 teaspoonful) • Children's melt-away tablets (80 mg) • Junior strength melt-away tablets (160 mg) • Rectal suppositories (available in many different amounts)	• As of mid-2011, infants' liquid is the same concentration (strength) as children's liquid, although they are available as different products. • Note different strengths of children's and junior tablets. • Be careful using suppositories, and don't cut them. • Acetaminophen can be an ingredient in many other over-the-counter products and may be abbreviated as "APAP." • Store safely to prevent accidental poisoning.
Ibuprofen • Motrin • Advil • generic	• Give amount by weight—this is more accurate than by age. • 5–10 mg per kilogram or 2.5–4.5 mg per pound of body weight.	• Every 6–8 hours; no more than 4 doses in 24 hours.	• Infants' suspension (50 mg per 1.25 ml) • Children's suspension (100 mg per 5 ml 1 teaspoonful) • Children's chewable tablet (50 mg) • Junior strength chewable tablet (100 mg) • Swallow tablets (200 mg)	• Do not give to infants less than 6 months of age. • Note different concentrations of infants' and children's liquids; infants' suspension is more concentrated (more mg in 1 ml). • Note different strengths of children's and junior tablets. • May last longer than acetaminophen—up to 8 hours. • Store safely to prevent accidental poisoning.

for each drug—children's and junior strength. The junior strength tablets have twice as much medicine in each tablet as the children's tablets. If you are not sure what strength tablet or liquid you are giving to your child, it is possible that you may give too much or too little medicine. Always look carefully at what product you are using before deciding how many tablets to give your child. If you are not sure what strength you are giving, don't hesitate to call your pharmacy. And don't hesitate to ask a pharmacist before buying medicine, to be sure that you are buying the right medicine for your child.

You can buy acetaminophen as a rectal suppository. Ibuprofen does not come as a suppository. Suppositories can be useful when a child has a fever and is vomiting and can't keep a liquid down. However, be extra careful when using rectal acetaminophen suppositories, as they may be absorbed into the bloodstream differently from liquid and tablets and may cause serious side effects. Be sure to speak with your pharmacist or doctor before using these suppositories. Acetaminophen suppositories come in many different strengths, which may be confusing. Do not cut a suppository in half or into quarters to use less, as the amount of medicine in these suppositories may not be spread out evenly.

You can buy both acetaminophen and ibuprofen as trade-name products—Tylenol for acetaminophen and Motrin or Advil for ibuprofen—and as generic products. The trade-name and generic products differ mainly by cost. Some trade-name products may be much more expensive than generic products. I believe that the trade products and the generics work equally well. Trade-name and generic products may differ by taste. Some of the trade-name products may taste better than the generics (which I found out when my son was young, as I relate in chapter 2). You may have to experiment to find out what product and flavor your child likes. Now that my children can swallow tablets, I always buy generic ibuprofen or acetaminophen for my family and myself.

---

*

Acetaminophen and ibuprofen come as many different products for infants and children. They differ in how much medicine they each contain. Be sure that you are using the right product, which has the right amount of medicine in it, for your child's weight and age.

*Which medication—acetaminophen or ibuprofen—is safer to use for
my child? I remember news stories about how dangerous Tylenol can be.
Is Tylenol dangerous for children?*

In 2009, acetaminophen (Tylenol) was in the national news. This
was because the Food and Drug Administration (FDA) met to discuss
new information about how dangerous acetaminophen may be. *If
too much acetaminophen is given*, it may damage a child's or an adult's
liver. The FDA discussed two medical studies of liver damage from
acetaminophen in adults and children. These studies found that acetaminophen is the main cause of liver damage in adults and the
second most common cause in children.

Both acetaminophen and ibuprofen are safe *when they are used correctly*. In this case, *correctly* means giving the right dose of medicine
for your child's weight and not giving medication more often than
instructed—no more than every 4 to 6 hours for acetaminophen and
no more than every 6 to 8 hours for ibuprofen. Children have died
from being given too much acetaminophen. Many of the parents of
these children were confused about the different products and accidentally gave too much medicine.

Ibuprofen is also a safe medicine when it is used correctly, but it
may cause some side effects. Ibuprofen can cause bleeding in the
stomach and an ulcer. However, this side effect rarely happens in
children. If your child has no medical conditions other than a fever
and has not had an ulcer before, it would be very unlikely for your
child to have stomach bleeding from ibuprofen. Ulcers from ibuprofen are much more likely to occur in adults, especially older adults.
Another side effect to consider is the possibility that ibuprofen may
damage the kidneys. This is more likely to happen if your child is dehydrated, which may occur with fever. With dehydration, less blood
goes to the kidneys, and ibuprofen may reduce the amount of blood
the kidneys get even further.

Ibuprofen (Motrin, Advil) became available as a children's liquid
product without a doctor's prescription (over the counter) in 1995.
A large medical study of more than 84,000 children showed that
ibuprofen given to children was not more likely to cause bleeding in

the stomach or intestines or to damage a child's kidneys as compared to acetaminophen (Tylenol).

Unless your child has other health conditions and your doctor has told you not to use ibuprofen, you can consider ibuprofen safe to give your child. If your child is not drinking or is vomiting, or if he or she has another medical condition that affects the kidneys, acetaminophen is probably a safer drug to use.

Acetaminophen is very safe when given in a correct amount. It has very few side effects, including (rarely) causing nausea. Most infants and children experience no side effects when given acetaminophen. However, and this is a big "however," acetaminophen may make your child very ill, and it may even kill your child, if too much is given. How could this happen? For example, if a young child, such as a 2-year-old, finds a bottle of acetaminophen liquid or chewable tablets and drinks or eats all the medicine in the bottle, the overdose or accidental poisoning could be deadly. (See Appendix C for ways to prevent accidental poisonings.) Be sure to place the child-resistant top back on the acetaminophen bottle every time you use it, and be sure to keep the bottle in a safe place. Another way acetaminophen can be dangerous or even deadly is if a parent or caregiver mistakenly gives a child too much medicine by using a wrong dosage form of acetaminophen, as I explain above.

What are some ways a parent might give the wrong amount of acetaminophen to their child?

The following four *wrong* ways of giving acetaminophen to a child could cause injury or even death. *Do not do these things.*

1. A parent may accidentally use tablets with more acetaminophen in them, such as junior strength or even adult tablets, for a young child.

2. More than one parent, or caregiver, may give medicine to a child without realizing that someone else already gave medicine.

3. A parent may give too much acetaminophen, or give it too often,

in the mistaken belief that "more is better." A parent may be tempted to give more medicine if his or her child's temperature doesn't come down to 98.6°F after giving medicine.

4. A parent may unknowingly give acetaminophen that is "hidden" in other over-the-counter products—especially in cough and cold products—in addition to giving acetaminophen for fever. Many over-the-counter products have acetaminophen in them, although this may not be clear on the product package.

Avoid these four common mistakes.

*

> Both acetaminophen and ibuprofen are safe when used correctly. Acetaminophen, however, can be dangerous if it is used incorrectly. To use acetaminophen and ibuprofen safely for your child, be sure you are giving the right amount and using the right type (dosage form) of medicine. When you are done giving each dose to your child, store the medicine in a safe place.

What common problems do parents have giving acetaminophen and ibuprofen to their children?

As discussed above, because these medicines come in so many different types, giving acetaminophen or ibuprofen may be confusing, and it is far too easy to give too much or too little to children. Several medical studies have tested how accurately parents give fever medicine to their children. In one study, the researchers asked parents to determine a correct amount of acetaminophen for their child. The parents were told their child's weight and were then given a bottle of acetaminophen liquid medicine and several measuring devices, such as a medicine spoon or dosing syringe. Only 40 percent of the parents were able to calculate a correct amount of acetaminophen, and only 30 percent were able both to calculate a correct dose and to measure the liquid dose correctly.

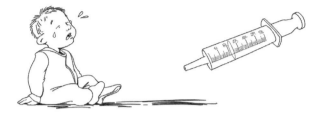

You want to help your child feel better. An oral dosing syringe with dosing lines can help you give him just the right amount of fever-reducing medication—no more and no less than is recommended for his age and size.

Other common problems parents may have with giving these medicines to their children include:

- Assuming that the dosage cup that comes with children's liquid medicine is supposed to be filled all the way to the top for all children.
- Using a kitchen teaspoon for giving a teaspoonful of medicine. Kitchen teaspoons are not accurate. Parents should always use medicine dosing spoons or dosing syringes to give liquid medicine to a child. (See chapter 2 for more about how to measure out liquid medicine.)

How to Calculate How Much Medicine to Give a Child

• •

Here is an example of how to give acetaminophen and ibuprofen correctly for an infant with a fever who is uncomfortable because of the fever.

Example: Your 10-month-old infant son has a fever of 102.5°F and weighs 22 pounds, or 10 kilograms (kg). You have spoken with your child's doctor, and she recommends giving acetaminophen or ibuprofen.

continued

ACETAMINOPHEN (TYLENOL OR GENERIC)

1. *How much acetaminophen should I give?*

- By weight ➡ 10–15 mg per kg or 4.5–6.5 mg per pound = 100–150 mg

- By age from medication box ➡ box says, "Ask a Doctor" ➡ the doctor's office will also tell you to give 100–150 mg.

2. *What type of acetaminophen should I use?*
   You can use either infants' liquid suspension or children's liquid suspension, as they are both the same concentration (strength). The infants' liquid comes with an oral syringe to help measure out a correct dose. An appropriate dose would be 3 to 4.5 ml. If you use the children's liquid suspension product, use an oral dosing syringe to measure out a correct dose (see chapter 2 for more about accurately measuring liquid medicines). Note that you may still have some of the older acetaminophen infants' drops in your home. Most acetaminophen infants' drops products were taken off pharmacy shelves in 2011 to try to reduce confusion between two different acetaminophen liquid products. This older infants' drops product is more concentrated—it has 80 mg in 0.8 ml. You can still use infants' drops if the medicine is not expired. Be careful, however, as the volume dose will be different from using the children's liquid. Call your pharmacist for help on how much to give.

3. *How should I measure out the amount to give?*
   Use an amount of medicine that will be easy, and accurate, to measure. The new infants' liquid product contains a dosing syringe with four different markings for four different doses—use the 3.75 ml marking, which is 120 mg. You can also use a regular dosing syringe to measure out 4 ml, which is 128 mg. This amount is about the same as ¾ of a teaspoon.

4. *How often should I give acetaminophen?*
   Acetaminophen can be given every 4 to 6 hours, but do not give acetaminophen to your child more than 5 times in a 24-hour period.

5. How do I know if acetaminophen is helping?

Watch your child's comfort level. He should begin feeling better within 30 to 60 minutes. Don't focus too much on his temperature, as it may not come down all the way to 98.6°F. If your son's temperature comes down to 99.5°F, and he feels better, then the medicine has helped.

6. How much should the fever come down?

Don't expect your child's temperature necessarily to come down to 98.6°F with fever medicine. For your son in this case, you could expect his temperature to come down to about 99.5°F to 100°F. Remember, making your child more comfortable is the main goal of treating his fever. Lowering his temperature to 98.6°F is not the main goal.

• •

IBUPROFEN (MOTRIN, ADVIL, OR GENERIC)

1. How much ibuprofen should I give?

- By weight ➡ 5-10 mg per kg or 2.5-4.5 mg per pound = 55-100 mg

- By directions from medication box:
    - 18-23 pounds ➡ 1.875 ml (third line on dropper) or 75 mg
    - 6-11 months ➡ 1.25 ml (second line on dropper) or 50 mg

- Notice that different doses are given by age and weight. Both doses may be correct, but 75 mg is in the middle of the correct range amount and is more likely to be effective, and 50 mg is on the low end of the range amount.

2. What type of ibuprofen should I use?

Use "infants' oral suspension" because it is more concentrated than children's suspension. You will give less liquid than if you used the children's suspension, which will be less likely to cause choking.

3. How should I measure out the amount to give?

- The dropper for infants' oral suspension has three lines on it. One line at 0.625 ml (25 mg), a second line at 1.25 ml (50 mg), and a third line at 1.875 ml (75 mg). A "dropperful" is considered up to the third line.

continued

- Use an amount that is easy to measure—50-100 mg is a correct dose as we determined. Thus 1.25 ml, 1.875 ml, or 2.50 ml (2 doses of 1.25 ml) are all correct. One dose at 75 mg (1.875 ml) is probably the easiest dose to give, as it is easy to measure and it is in the middle of the correct range.

- If your child is very uncomfortable, and you want to give the maximum amount of medicine (100 mg) use two droppersful of 1.25 ml each.

4. How often should I give ibuprofen?

Ibuprofen may be given every 6 to 8 hours, but do not give ibuprofen to your child more than 4 times in a 24-hour period.

5. How do I know if ibuprofen is helping?

Watch your child's comfort level. He should begin feeling better within 30 to 60 minutes. Don't focus too much on his temperature, as it may not come down all the way to 98.6°F. If your son's temperature comes down to 99.5°F, and he feels better, then the medicine has helped.

6. How much should the fever come down?

Don't expect your child's temperature to always come down to 98.6°F with fever medicine. In this case, you could expect his temperature to come down to about 99.5-100°F. Remember, making your child more comfortable is the main goal of treating his fever, not lowering his temperature to 98.6°F.

• • • • • • •

This example shows how complicated it can be to calculate the correct dose of acetaminophen or ibuprofen to give your infant or child and how easy it can be to make an error in the calculation. You may also have questions about which product to use and how to measure out the correct dose. If you are not sure, don't guess. Instead, ask your pharmacist or doctor for help.

CHAPTER 4

How Do I Use Medicines for Infection?

In this chapter I discuss medicines given to infants and children to treat infections. Most children have many infections throughout childhood, for a variety of reasons described in this chapter. It is best to use antibiotics to treat infection only when they are necessary. This is not because antibiotics are unsafe but because the more often we use antibiotics, the more likely the bacteria (germs) that cause infections will become resistant to antibiotics. *Resistance* means that the bacteria mutate, or change in a way that makes antibiotics ineffective in killing them. An infection caused by an antibiotic-resistant germ is harder to treat; a child suffering from this kind of infection may require additional antibiotics that have more side effects or may even need hospitalization.

When it comes to infections, you may wonder:

- Why does my son get so many ear infections? Does he always need an antibiotic?

- What is the best antibiotic for my son's infection?

- Does my daughter always need an antibiotic for a fever or cough?

- My daughter has thick, disgusting snot coming out of her nose. Does she need an antibiotic?

- My son has a very sore throat, but his doctor said he doesn't need an antibiotic. Why not?

- My daughter has the flu. Does she need an antibiotic?

- Are all of the antibiotics prescribed for my son safe for him?

- My daughter is always getting sick with infections.
  Is there anything I can do to prevent this?

Infection is a very common reason parents take their children to see a doctor. National surveys show that children are frequently seen in a doctor's office for infections, including otitis media (ear infections), pharyngitis (sore throat), respiratory infections (such as the common cold and sinus infections), and others. Infants and children may develop many other types of infections as well. Skin infections, respiratory infections (for example, nose, ears, lungs), and gastrointestinal tract infections (such as diarrhea) are among the most common. Fortunately, most of these infections can be treated and cured. More serious (and potentially deadly) infections in infants and children include meningitis (infection of the brain), pertussis (whooping cough), pneumonia, and influenza (the "flu"). Vaccines may prevent or reduce the seriousness of some of these infections. (See chapter 5 for more information about vaccines.)

Infants and children may have fevers, coughs, or diarrhea when they have an infection. The term *germ* is used here to describe small organisms that can cause infection in humans. Infection is caused by bacteria, viruses, fungi, and parasites, any of which may also be called a "germ." Viruses and bacteria are responsible for many of the infections in infants and children. The type of medicine a child may need depends on the type of germ causing an infection.

Viruses generally do not require treatment with a specific medicine. The common infections of infants and children, such as colds and sore throats, are often caused by viruses for which there is no specific medicine. There are a few viral infections, however, that can be treated with specific antiviral medicines. The best example is influenza, the "flu." (See later in this chapter for more about the flu.)

Sometimes doctors are not able to identify what type of germ is causing a child's infection. A child's symptoms (how he or she feels) help the doctor identify what is causing the infection. Medicine often is useful in treating symptoms, such as a stuffy nose or fever, but the medicine does not need to be an antibiotic. When viruses cause infection in infants and children, antibiotics are not helpful and are not needed. This is a very important point: *antibiotics are often not necessary because viruses cause many infections, and antibiotics do not kill viruses.*

Ask your child's doctor if a virus or a bacteria is causing your child's infection. Viruses can cause infection and make your child feel ill, with fever, cough, runny mucus or snot, or diarrhea. Common viruses include RSV (respiratory syncytial virus), rhinovirus and adenovirus (these cause the common cold), and rotavirus (which causes diarrhea).

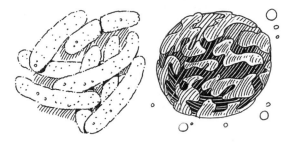

Microscopic bacteria and viruses cause infections.
Under a microscope they look something like this.

✳

Several types of germs cause infections in children. Viruses cause many infections in children, and antibiotics do not kill viruses. Bacteria cause some infections, and antibiotics can be helpful in killing the bacteria that are causing the infection. Not all childhood infections need to be treated with an antibiotic. Ask your child's doctor what is causing your child's infection and whether an antibiotic is necessary.

Why does my son get so many infections? What can I do to reduce the number of infections he gets?

Children often have more respiratory tract infections, such as the common cold, than adults. This happens because of several factors: children have a less mature immune system (for fighting infection) than adults do, children's hygiene habits are worse than adults' are, and children are more often exposed to other sick people than adults are (through child care or school). Most germs are passed among people by direct contact (by touching a person who is carrying the germs) or by indirect contact (by touching an object that has germs on it or being sneezed or coughed on). The more people that are in an area and the closer together they are (such as in child care or a classroom), the more likely it is that germs will be passed along.

Child care is a major reason why children get infections so often. With both parents often working full-time or part-time out of the home, it is now common for young children to be in some type of child care. Several studies have shown that children in child care are more likely to catch respiratory infections such as colds, ear infections, sore throats, and pneumonias. For example, in one study of 2,568 children from 1 to 7 years of age, children in child care had an increased risk of having more colds, ear infections, and pneumonias, as compared to children not in child care. Children in a smaller, family child care, such as private child care in a person's home, were not more likely to develop these infections in this study. Other studies have also shown that children younger than 2 years of age who attend child care are much more likely to have ear infections and that the risk increases in larger child care centers. Ear infections (otitis media) are the most common reason overall why children use antibiotics. Several studies have shown that children in child care generally receive more antibiotics (and not just for ear infections)—2 to 3 times more antibiotics as compared to children at home, according to some studies. Studies have also shown that children in child care are more likely to have infections with germs resistant to antibiotics, which are harder to treat. Children with infections caused by resistant germs are also more likely to be sicker.

Frequent exposure to tobacco smoking is another cause of increased risk of infection for children. Infants who are not breast-fed in the first year of life are at increased risk for some types of infections. And of course, not immunizing your child with the routine pediatric immunizations, including influenza, is a major factor for increasing the risk of your child developing infections, many of which could kill your child. (See chapter 5 for more information about vaccines.)

As a parent, what can you do to reduce the risk of infection in your child? Here are several steps you and your family can take:

Smoking
Cut back on how much you smoke, or, better, stop smoking. I hear many parents say, "I don't smoke in front of my children," or "I smoke outside." Studies have shown that these precautions don't much matter because the smoke and particles and tobacco smell remain on clothing, in hair, and throughout the house.

Child care
Because attending larger child care centers may increase the chance that your child will have more infections, placing your child in a smaller child care center may reduce the number of infections. Removing a child from child care may not be possible if both parents work. If your child stays in child care, talk to the child care workers about their hygiene policies and insist that they follow recommendations from your state health department and the Centers for Disease Control and Prevention, an agency of the federal government.

Good personal hygiene
Good personal hygiene is one of the best measures for preventing or reducing the number of infections your child gets. Hand washing is the single most effective way you can prevent or reduce infections. Clean your hands before eating, after using the bathroom, after blowing your nose, and before preparing food.

Your child, you, and everyone in your home needs to practice good hand washing. What is "good" hand washing? Use soap and water and wash hands for at least 15 to 20 seconds. This is important. Most people don't use enough soap or wash for long enough. One way to know if you are washing long enough is to sing "Happy Birthday to You" *twice* while washing.

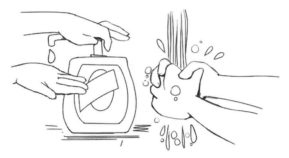

Careful hand washing and using alcohol gel to clean hands may help prevent infection.

Many soaps, especially liquid soaps, are sold as "antibacterial." Most of these antibacterial soaps contain a chemical called triclosan. Studies have shown that triclosan is no more effective than plain soap at cleaning hands, and some scientists have concerns about triclosan possibly increasing antibiotic resistance. The Food and Drug Administration stated in 2005 that antibacterial soaps are no more effective than plain soaps.

Good hygiene habits in the home also include cleaning shared items and surfaces, especially if someone is ill with an infection. If soap and water are not available, use an alcohol-based hand gel. Carry alcohol-based hand gels with you in your purse and car, and use them when soap and water aren't available. You need to use alcohol-based hand gel generously: put gel on your hands and your child's hands and rub those hands together for 10 to 15 seconds. If your hands are totally dry after 10 seconds, you didn't put on enough gel. One study that looked at families regularly using alcohol-based hand gels with at least one child in child care showed that they had fewer respiratory tract infections, such as the common cold, than families not using alcohol-based hand gels. A word of caution about alcohol-based hand gels, however: because they contain a lot of alcohol (ethyl alcohol)—more alcohol than in whiskey—they may be dangerous if young children accidentally ingest them. When you are done using them, store them in a safe place.

Immunizations

Adhering to the immunization schedule recommended for children is the best way to prevent common and dangerous infections. See chapter 5 for more information on immunizations.

Breast-feeding

Breast-feeding in the first year of life has been shown to reduce some types of infections in infants. Human breast milk contains substances that can reduce ear infections, diarrhea, pneumonia, and meningitis, among others.

*

> Children often have more infections than adults, and children use more antibiotics than adults. Parents can reduce the chance of infection occurring in their children by practicing good personal hygiene, using smaller child care centers, stopping or reducing smoking, and most importantly, having children immunized.

My 5-year-old son has a fever of 100.5°F and a runny nose. I took him to our pediatrician, who said that my son does not need an antibiotic. Why not? Why shouldn't he get an antibiotic?

Our society is comfortable receiving an antibiotic when someone has a fever or "has an infection." In fact, we often expect to receive an antibiotic whenever someone is sick. It's common for younger children to have a cold about once a month, and some parents believe that an antibiotic is always or frequently necessary to treat these colds. Viruses, and not bacteria, cause many fevers and snotty noses in children. Antibiotics kill bacteria, not viruses. Snot coming from your son's nose has nothing to do with needing an antibiotic. Snot, even if it is green, thick, and gross-looking, is made up of dead cells that are destroyed by the infection. Viruses and bacteria both can cause a child's nose to have a lot of snot.

Medical professionals use the term *antibiotic* to mean medicine used to treat infection caused by bacteria, not infection caused by the many other types of germs, such as viruses, fungi, parasitic worms, or protozoans. Medicines are available to treat some types infections caused by these other germs, but they are called by different names: antiviral, antifungal, antiparasitic (antihelmintic), or antiprotozoal medicines. Antibiotics are among the most commonly used medicines in children, and children receive more antibiotics than adults, as children have more infections than adults. Some of the more commonly used antibiotics in children are amoxicillin, Augmentin, and Zithromax.

Consider asking your child's doctor the following questions about whether your child needs to take an antibiotic:

- What type of germ is causing my child's infection? Is it a virus or bacteria? Or is it another type of germ that an antibiotic or similar type of medicine, such as an antifungal medicine, may help? (This is the most important question to ask because viruses cause most infections in infants and children, and antibiotics are not necessary to treat viral infections.)

- If antibiotics can't help, then what medicines will help relieve my child's symptoms and make him or her feel better?

Don't pressure your child's doctor to prescribe an antibiotic. Several studies have shown that some doctors are more likely to prescribe an antibiotic when parents pressure them to do so, even if the doctor believes that an antibiotic is not necessary for the child.

My 12-month-old daughter has been fussy, and I took her to our pediatrician. He told me that she has an ear infection and needs an antibiotic, and he gave me a prescription. Is this the best antibiotic for her? It's a different antibiotic from the last one that she was given for an ear infection. Why?

Doctors have many different choices when prescribing an antibiotic (table 4.1). Several factors help your doctor decide which antibiotic is best for your daughter for this ear infection (acute otitis media). Perhaps most important is the type of infection and the types of germs that are most likely causing the infection. Other important factors include:

- your daughter's age,
- the symptoms your daughter has now and how sick she is,
- whether the antibiotic is available as a liquid (for a 12-month-old child, a liquid would be best),
- any allergies to medicine your daughter may have,
- other medical conditions she may have,
- what type of medication insurance you have (because some antibiotics may not be covered by your insurance plan and could be much more expensive for you),
- the date of your daughter's most recent antibiotic (a recently used antibiotic may cause the germs for this infection to be more resistant to some antibiotics), and
- whether your daughter attends child care.

The specific types of germs that cause an ear infection for a 12-month-old child are well known to pediatricians. The ear infection and the symptoms your daughter has now may be different from her last infection, and a different antibiotic may be best for her now.

Yesterday our pediatrician prescribed the antibiotic amoxicillin to treat my 12-month-old daughter's ear infection. I've given it to her twice, but her ears still seem to be hurting. What can I give her for this ear pain?

Amoxicillin is often the best antibiotic for children with ear infections. It works well; it tastes good; it is safe; and it is inexpensive. It

TABLE 4.1 Commonly used antibiotics for infants and children

GENERIC NAME	TRADE NAME	HOW OFTEN TO GIVE	MOST COMMON SIDE EFFECTS	GIVE WITH OR WITHOUT FOOD?	LIQUID TASTE	NEED TO REFRIGERATE?	COMMENTS
Amoxicillin	Amoxil	Usually twice a day (every 8–12 hours)	Loose stools, diarrhea, rash	With or without food	Good: bubble gum, fruit, mixed berry	Not necessary, but refrigeration may improve taste.	• OK to mix with milk, formula, or juice for infants. • Also available as chewable tablets.
Amoxicillin-clavulanate	Augmentin	Usually twice a day (every 8–12 hours.	Loose stools, diarrhea, rash	With food	Good: orange, strawberry cream, orange raspberry	Refrigerate.	• OK to mix with milk, formula, or juice for infants. • Also available as chewable tablets.
Cefuroxime axetil	Ceftin	Twice a day	Loose stools, diarrhea	Liquid: with food; tablets: with or without food	Not good: tutti-frutti	Refrigerate.	• Don't crush tablets or they will have a bitter taste. • Pharmacy can add flavors to improve taste.
Cefprozil	Cefzil	Twice a day	Loose stools, diarrhea	With or without food	Good: bubble gum, tutti-frutti	Refrigerate.	

Medication	Brand	Frequency	Side effects	Food	Taste	Refrigeration	Notes
Cefdinir	Omnicef	Once or twice a day	Loose stools, diarrhea	With or without food	Good: strawberry, cherry	Do not refrigerate liquid as it may make very thick.	• Do not give with iron, vitamins with iron, or antacids. • OK to mix with iron-fortified infant formula.
Cefpodoxime proxetil	Vantin	Twice a day	Loose stools, diarrhea	Liquid: with or without food; tablet: with food	Not good: lemon crème, fruit	Refrigerate.	• Pharmacy can add flavors to improve taste.
Clindamycin palmitate	Cleocin	Three to four times a day	Loose stools, diarrhea (may be severe and dangerous)	With or without food	Not good: cherry	Do not refrigerate liquid as it may make very thick.	• Has bad taste; pharmacy may be able to improve taste with added flavoring.
Cotrimoxazole (TMP-SMX)	Bactrim, Sulfatrim, Septra	Twice a day	Loose stools, rash (may be severe and dangerous)	With or without food	Fair: cherry	Not necessary, but refrigeration may improve taste.	• Pharmacy may be able to improve taste with added flavoring.

may take two or three days before amoxicillin begins to make your daughter's ear infection go away and for her to feel better. Ear infections can be very painful because a lot of fluid builds up behind the eardrum (tympanic membrane), putting pressure on the eardrum and parts of the ear, which can hurt.

You can give your daughter acetaminophen (Tylenol) or ibuprofen (Motrin or Advil) for pain. You can call your pediatrician or pharmacist, and they will tell you how much to give, based on your daughter's weight. Chapter 3 can help you figure out how much of either medicine to give your daughter, too.

There are other medicines that you can put into your daughter's ears to help relieve her pain, and these medicines work well. Several generic products containing benzocaine and antipyrine are available, but you will need a prescription from your pediatrician. These products contain two medicines that can reduce pain when put on the eardrum and skin in the ear. One product you can buy without a prescription in a pharmacy or health-food store is a natural herbal product that has been tested in a published medical study and was shown to work just as well as the prescription product with two anesthetic medicines. This herbal extract product contained garlic, mullein, Saint-John's-wort, and *Calendula flores* in olive oil. Health-food stores and some pharmacies may also carry other products similar to this natural ear oil product.

Is the new antibiotic my daughter's pediatrician prescribed safe for my daughter?

Fortunately, most antibiotics that are prescribed for infants and children are safe; overall, antibiotics are some of the safest medicines we have for children. As I discuss in chapter 1, however, all medicines have side effects. While several antibiotics may cause dangerous side effects in children, the antibiotics commonly given for ear infections in infants and children typically have few side effects, and these are usually minor. Of course, you should always ask your child's doctor about the side effects of the antibiotic that is prescribed.

The side effects most likely to occur for the commonly used antibiotics for ear infections include loose stools (stools that are not

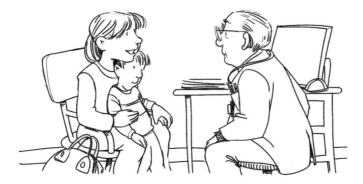

formed), diarrhea (mostly watery stools), nausea, abdominal cramps, or rash. Some children may develop a rash after taking an antibiotic, but this rash is usually not due to an allergy to the antibiotic (see below for more information about allergies to antibiotics).

Loose stools or diarrhea commonly occur with antibiotics because the antibiotics kill some of the natural "good" bacteria that live in a child's gastrointestinal tract (mouth, stomach, intestines). Many, many good bacteria live in our gastrointestinal tract; these bacteria are good because they serve many useful purposes, such as keeping out "bad" bacteria, and because they help to metabolize (chemically change) and digest chemicals and foods. When these good bacteria are killed, the normal process of forming stool may change, resulting in loose stools or diarrhea.

Some children often develop loose stools from antibiotics, while other children rarely or never experience this side effect. If loose stools develop, it is usually not serious or something to be overly concerned about. Most courses of antibiotics are 5 to 10 days long; once the antibiotic therapy is finished, your child's normal stool pattern should return. What may be worrisome is if diarrhea develops and the child loses a lot of fluid. The diarrhea is not usually a problem, but the fluid loss may be a concern because infants and children can easily become dehydrated. If your child develops loose stools or especially watery diarrhea while receiving an antibiotic, you should call your child's doctor. It is a good idea always to keep oral rehydration solution (one common trade name is Pedialyte) on hand because an oral rehydration solution usually should be given to your child if she becomes dehydrated. (See chapter 6 for more information about oral rehydration solutions.) If your child has blood or mucus in her stools or severe abdominal pain or cramps, it could be a potentially serious side effect from antibiotics called antibiotic-associated diarrhea and you should call her doctor immediately. Fortunately, antibiotic-associated diarrhea does not commonly occur with most antibiotics.

If your child develops loose stools or diarrhea from an antibiotic, it may be useful to try to replace the good intestinal bacteria by giving her a probiotic. A probiotic is good bacteria in a medicine-like form (such as a capsule or tablet). You can purchase probiotics in health-food stores and many pharmacies. One product that is likely to help is called Culturelle. It is not typically necessary to give probiotics to all children to prevent loose stools or diarrhea from an antibiotic. However, if your child needs an antibiotic and frequently has had loose stools or diarrhea from antibiotics, giving a probiotic with the antibiotic to prevent diarrhea may be helpful. Some yogurts contain probiotic bacteria (advertised as "live and active cultures"). Don't rely on yogurts for this use, however, because they probably do not contain enough of the probiotic bacteria to replace what an antibiotic kills. Use the product Culturelle instead.

Most antibiotics are safe, and their most common side effects are usually not dangerous. Because antibiotics are so commonly used in children, these side effects, although not usually dangerous, may still be a problem. A 2008 study looked at children and adults who went to one of 63 hospital emergency rooms in the United States in 2004, 2005, and 2006 because of a side effect from a medicine. Of all these visits to an emergency room because of a side effect from any type of medicine, 19.3 percent were due to side effects from an antibiotic. This equals 142,505 emergency room visits (by both adults and children) over three years because of a side effect from an antibiotic. Children (14 years of age and younger) had 25.9 percent of the total emergency room visits, and the rate of side effects was highest among children younger than 12 months. Antibiotic side effects, even though they usually aren't dangerous, are one reason it's best to use antibiotics only when they are necessary.

Most antibiotics given to children for common infections have minor side effects. Loose stools or diarrhea is the most common side effect, and it is usually not dangerous. Watery diarrhea may lead to dehydration, however. You should keep oral rehydration solutions at home in case your child develops diarrhea from antibiotics. Antibiotics should be used only when your child has an infection caused by bacteria.

My daughter is 26 months old and has been fussy for the past 24 hours. I took her to our pediatrician, and he told us she might have an ear infection, although he was not sure. He said that she doesn't need an antibiotic, at least not now. Why? Shouldn't all children with an ear infection get an antibiotic?

Not all children may need an antibiotic for an ear infection, at least not right away. In 2004 the American Academy of Pediatrics came out with recommendations that not all children with an ear infection need an antibiotic. Why? Many ear infections can go away without an antibiotic, as the body's immune system helps cure the infection. Not using an antibiotic initially is called "observation." This means that the child is closely watched for up to 72 hours after she becomes ill. If she is improving, then an antibiotic is probably not necessary. If she has not improved, then the doctor will prescribe an antibiotic. Because not all children may need an antibiotic for an ear infection (and in some cases the child may not in fact have an ear infection), this "observation" period reduces the amount of antibiotics a child uses.

For some infants and children, it may be difficult for a doctor to accurately determine if a true ear infection is present. An infant or child with a common cold may have ear pain and symptoms similar to a true ear infection. There are specific factors that doctors use (such as the appearance of the tympanic membrane, or ear drum) to determine accurately if a true infection is present, and an infant or child may show some, but not all, of these factors. Observation also reduces cost, potential side effects from the antibiotic, and perhaps most important, the chance that resistant germs will develop in the child.

Only certain children should be considered for observation. For example, infants younger than 6 months of age and infants or children with a severe ear infection (high fever or severe ear pain) should receive an antibiotic immediately. Your daughter, because she is older than 24 months, may be observed first. The pediatrician may also decide not to use antibiotics right away if she believes that your daughter's ear infection is "non-severe," which means that she has a fever of less than 102°F and her ear pain is mild. Also, she may not prescribe an antibiotic if she isn't sure that your daughter actually has an ear infection. The child may just have a cold, not an ear infection. If the doctor is sure that a child has an ear infection, then antibiotics should be used because they are helpful. Two studies published in 2011 showed that antibiotics are helpful when an infant or child actually does have a true ear infection. During observation we always treat a child's pain and discomfort—we *never* recommend *not* using acetaminophen (Tylenol) or ibuprofen (Motrin or Advil) to help the child feel better. But in the case of antibiotics, we wait a few days to see if the child will get better on her own, without an antibiotic.

If antibiotics are usually safe to use, why shouldn't I ask my doctor to prescribe an antibiotic for my son when he is sick or has a high fever?

Even though antibiotics are mostly safe for children, giving them to children can cause another problem. Unnecessary courses of antibiotics may help bacteria become resistant to the antibiotics' killing effects. If your child's infection is caused by a strain of antibiotic-resistant bacteria, many antibiotics may not work for that infection. Such infections may become severe and spread to other parts of your child's body, which can be serious. The more often antibiotics are given to a child, the more likely it is that bacteria will become resistant to the antibiotics.

Antibiotic resistance is a major health problem in the United States. Bacteria become resistant to antibiotics in several ways, depending on the type of bacteria and the type of antibiotic. An antibiotic will kill the bacteria that are sensitive to it. However, among the millions of bacteria, a few of them will not be killed. The surviving bacteria are naturally more resistant to the antibiotic. These bacteria then multiply, and before long, millions of antibiotic-resistant bacteria are alive. When these bacteria cause an infection, it is more difficult to treat, and fewer antibiotics are available to combat them. Antibiotic-resistant bacteria can also spread to other children in your family, or to you, and cause infection. Many infections caused by resistant bacteria have to be treated with more expensive antibiotics, which may have more side effects. This is another reason for your child not to have a lot of antibiotics.

What can you do to prevent antibiotic-resistant bacteria from causing an infection in your child? Perhaps most importantly, don't demand an antibiotic when you take your child to see a doctor. Viruses cause many infections in children, and antibiotics don't kill viruses. Ask your child's doctor whether a virus or bacteria is causing your child's infection. If an antibiotic is necessary for your child, be sure to use it exactly as directed by your doctor and pharmacist. If any of the antibiotic is left over, don't save it for "next time." Throw away any extra antibiotic.

My 18-month-old son has been taking amoxicillin for three days for an ear infection. Now he has a rash on his chest. Is he allergic to amoxicillin?

Because antibiotics are used so often in infants and children, parents may say that their child is "allergic" to a specific antibiotic because he gets a rash. I put "allergic" in quotation marks because many parents, and even some doctors, misuse the word *allergy*. When a parent says that his child is "allergic" to an antibiotic, often what actually happened was that the child experienced a side effect from the medicine, such as diarrhea, stomach cramps, or drowsiness.

Many people call these side effects, or any unwanted effect from an antibiotic, an "allergy." These effects are not likely a real medication allergy, according to the medical definition of *allergy*. There are four general types of allergies to medications. The type that doctors most worry about is called *anaphylaxis*. Anaphylaxis is a very quick

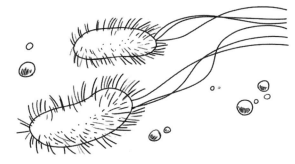

Antibiotics are used to kill bacteria that are causing infection.
Bacteria are shown as they might look under a microscope.

reaction to a medicine that causes a person to have trouble breathing or to lose consciousness. It can be very dangerous. It is unlikely for most children to have an anaphylactic reaction when taking a medicine.

Changes that may indicate that your child is having an allergic reaction include a rash that looks like hives (large raised, swollen bumps on the skin) or a rash that is itchy. If your child has difficulty breathing soon after taking a medicine, this is likely a dangerous allergic reaction, and you should call for help immediately. Also look for a swollen tongue or lips as a sign that a real allergy is occurring.

What is confusing is that many children develop rashes that look similar to those caused by a medication allergy, but these rashes usually are not allergic reactions. The rashes can look like small, red spots or small bumps (not like larger hives and often not very itchy). Infections from viruses commonly cause rashes in children, called *viral exanthems*. Antibiotics can also cause these rashes (but they are not true allergic, or anaphylactic, rashes). Up to 13 percent of children taking amoxicillin develop these rashes that are not due to a true, anaphylactic allergy.

Penicillin and similar antibiotics (such as amoxicillin) cause true allergies more commonly than other antibiotics, and many people claim that they are "allergic" to penicillin. There have been several studies to determine if people who say that they are "allergic" to penicillin truly are allergic. Penicillin is the only antibiotic for which someone can be tested for a true allergy, by skin testing. If someone has a positive skin test for penicillin allergy, then he or she has a high risk of having a serious allergic reaction to penicillin and should not take it. In these studies, 80 to 90 percent of those claiming an "allergy" to penicillin did not have a positive skin test; they were not really allergic to penicillin.

What should you do if a rash develops on your son's chest after three days of taking amoxicillin? Certainly, call your son's doctor to discuss the rash. Tell the doctor what it looks like and whether it is bothering your son. It is possible that this rash is caused by a true allergy to amoxicillin, but it is much more likely that there is another cause for the rash. It could be a viral rash, an allergy to something else your son was exposed to, or another type of rash from amoxicillin that is not due to an anaphylaxis allergy.

Depending on what the rash looks like and whether it is bothering your son, the doctor may want to continue the course of amoxicillin for your son's infection. Stopping amoxicillin because of this rash, and stating that your son is allergic to amoxicillin (when he is not likely to be) can cause other problems. For one thing, it limits what antibiotics can be given to your son for future bacterial infections. It is likely that he will have many other infections throughout childhood. Amoxicillin is one of the most useful antibiotics we have for children: it kills many common bacteria, it is inexpensive, and liquid amoxicillin tastes good. There are also other antibiotics that are chemically similar to amoxicillin, and doctors may be afraid to use these antibiotics, as well, in a child with an "allergy" to amoxicillin. Doctors may then use different antibiotics that may not work as well to cure your child's infection.

So if your son does not have a proven allergy (anaphylaxis) to amoxicillin, it would be best not to say that he is "allergic" to it. If you want to find out if your son is truly allergic to penicillin (as noted, penicillin is the same chemical class as amoxicillin), a doctor specializing in allergies (allergist) can do a skin test with a specially made medicine.

This happened to my son. When he was about 3 years old, a doctor prescribed amoxicillin to him for an ear infection. At the same time, he had a viral infection that was giving him diarrhea. The day after taking the amoxicillin, he had a rash (not hives) on his chest. A

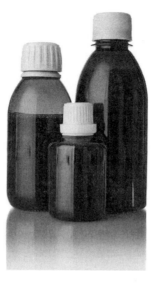

Medications commonly used for young children, such as antibiotics, are best given as liquids.

pediatrician told my wife and me that our son was allergic to amoxicillin. For my part, I wondered if the virus was causing the rash or if my son was really allergic to amoxicillin. I took him to an allergist, who gave him a skin test for penicillin allergy. The test was negative. After this, whenever I was asked if my son had any medication allergies, I would say no. If he had not been tested for a penicillin allergy, I would have had to say yes, and that would have limited the type of antibiotics he could take.

My 7-year-old daughter's doctor gave us a sample of Augmentin liquid for an ear infection, but he didn't give me many directions on how to use it. What is the correct way to give liquid antibiotics?

Augmentin (amoxicillin-clavulanate) is one of the more common antibiotics given to children for many types of infections. Augmentin is mostly used for the treatment of ear infections (see section above on ear infections). It is a very good antibiotic, as it can kill many types of bacteria that cause infection in children. As with any antibiotic, it will work best for your child if it is given correctly.

The following instructions should be followed when giving oral antibiotics to children:

- *Measure doses carefully.* Use an accurate dosing device, such as a dosing syringe, to measure out the liquid dose. (See chapter 2 for information about measuring liquid medicines.)

- *Finish the whole prescription.* Always finish the entire course of an antibiotic. Don't stop giving it as soon as your child is feeling better.

- *Space doses apart.* Augmentin is usually given twice a day. Give each dose at a time that is convenient for you, approximately every 8 to 12 hours. (The exact time is not critically important, and you don't need to disturb your child's sleep at night to give a dose.)

- *Follow label directions.* Give Augmentin exactly as stated on the bottle label, no more and no less, and not more or less often.

- *Shake.* Shake the bottle before pouring out each dose.

- *Store carefully.* Augmentin should be stored in the refrigerator to preserve its effectiveness. (Cold also improves the taste.)

- *Give with meals.* To reduce side effects such as diarrhea, Augmentin is best given with meals. A good time to give it is with breakfast and dinner.

My daughter seems to be sick so often, with ear infections and other types of infections. Our pharmacy is our second home! Even with health insurance, the cost of the all the antibiotics adds up. When she has some antibiotic left over, why can't I save it and use it for the next infection she gets?

Some antibiotics can be expensive; even with health insurance, the cost can easily add up when children frequently take antibiotics. It would be tempting to save any leftover antibiotic to use next time your child is ill with an infection. However, for several reasons, don't! For one thing, the antibiotic she is taking for this infection may not be the best antibiotic for the next infection. Your daughter's doctor needs to decide which antibiotic is the best treatment for each infection. Additionally, parents who save leftover antibiotic may give it to

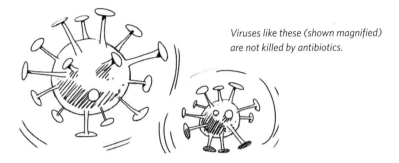

Viruses like these (shown magnified) are not killed by antibiotics.

their child when the child seems sick. But if the child's symptoms are due to a viral infection, the antibiotics won't help, and their overuse may lead to antibiotic resistance. This means that the next time your child has a bacterial infection, it may be harder to treat if antibiotic-resistant bacteria are causing it. It may take more antibiotics to knock out the infection, which increases the cost and the chances of side effects. Although it can be tempting to save any leftover antibiotic, it's best for your child for you to throw out the leftover antibiotic.

My 6-year-old daughter has a high fever, headache, coughing, and muscle aches. She began complaining of a bad headache, and she started coughing three days ago. Our doctor tested her for the flu, and the test was positive. Should she take an antibiotic? Are there medicines for the flu?

Influenza—the flu—is a viral infection of the respiratory system. With the flu, the respiratory system (nose, throat, lungs) is affected the most, but muscle aches, fever and chills, fatigue, headache, and lack of appetite are other symptoms. People with flu often feel bad all over. The most common symptoms of influenza in children are fever, cough, stuffy nose, headache, and sore throat. Influenza in children can also cause vomiting, diarrhea, and abdominal pain.

Many people confuse having the flu with having a cold. Parents may say that they or their children had the flu when it is more likely that they had a cold. What is the difference between the common cold and influenza? The common cold, like flu, is caused by viruses—in fact, over 200 different viruses can cause the common cold. Influenza is a much more serious viral infection than a cold, and children with the flu are sicker and feel much worse than children with a cold.

Colds mostly affect the upper respiratory tract—the nose, throat, eyes, and ears. Coughing from a cold and coughing from the flu differ. Coughing from a cold is not usually severe and can be productive, which means that mucus is coughed up. A child with a cold may feel congested when coughing. Coughing from the flu can be more painful and troublesome, and it is usually dry (little mucus is coughed up). Children with a cold often don't have a fever (medically, a fever is 100.5°F or higher), and if they do, it is usually not high. Children with a cold usually don't have other body symptoms, such as body aches. Young infants with a cold can have more breathing problems because the airways in their lungs are small and because young infants have trouble breathing through their mouths when their noses are stuffed up.

Influenza can be very dangerous. About 36,000 people die from the flu every year. Flu mostly causes death in elderly people, but some children die as well, although most of these children have other health problems that affect the lungs, heart, immune system, or nervous system. Between September 2010 and August 2011, 115 children died from the flu in the United States—53 of these children were younger than 5 years old. The majority of the children who died had *not* received a flu shot. Children don't die from the common cold.

Influenza is also often confused with the "stomach flu." When people say "stomach flu" they usually mean diarrhea or vomiting. Other types of viruses or bacteria may cause infections with symptoms mostly of nausea, vomiting, or diarrhea. While influenza may also cause these symptoms, it mostly affects the respiratory system, causing severe coughing and difficulty breathing. A specific virus—an influenza virus—causes influenza. There are three types of influenza viruses: A, B, and C. Influenza A more commonly causes illness in adults and children than influenza B or C. Influenza viruses mutate (change) frequently, which is why a new flu vaccine is needed each year. This is also why different years have different kinds of flu seasons, some worse than others. Influenza viruses in some years are more likely to make people sicker than the influenza viruses in other years.

During the 2009 influenza season, two types of influenza caused children and adults to be sick. These were called *seasonal influenza* and *H1N1 influenza*. H1N1 influenza was also called "swine flu" because some of the genes in this virus are similar to influenza viruses that normally occur in pigs. H1N1 influenza is the preferred term, however. Seasonal influenza is caused by other types of influenza viruses as well.

Parents of children of all ages—young infants to adolescents—should take influenza seriously because it can make children and adults very sick. Influenza often causes children to miss many days of school or child care, which may force parents to miss work to stay home with their sick child. Children have a higher influenza infection rate than adults; they are more likely to spread infection and become infected. Children younger than 5 years of age are hospitalized with influenza as often as adults aged 50 to 64 years. Children younger than 6 months of age and children 6 to 23 months of age are most likely to be hospitalized among all children and adolescents. Most children who die from influenza have some type of other health problem that affects the lungs, heart, immune system, or nervous system. Children who otherwise are healthy, however, can also die from influenza. Of the 115 children who died from influenza between 2010 and 2011, 56 had no other known medical problems.

How does your doctor know if your child has influenza? If your child is sick during influenza season (from October to April) with symptoms that look like influenza, then the doctor may assume your child has influenza. This assumption is often called a "clinical diagnosis," but it may not be accurate, as other viruses, such as RSV (respiratory syncytial virus), can cause similar symptoms, especially in infants. It is best if your child is tested for the influenza virus using a nose or throat swab. Results of these tests are often available within 30 minutes. A problem with some of these tests is that they may not be sensitive enough—even if the test is negative, your child may have influenza. If influenza has been documented in your community, these tests may not be necessary. It is important to know what is causing your child's illness. If influenza is the cause, the doctor can prescribe appropriate medicines, and others, such as antibiotics, can be avoided.

Because a virus causes the flu, antibiotics usually are not necessary. Sometimes children and adults with influenza have secondary bacterial infections of the lungs—pneumonia. Pneumonia makes children very sick, with painful breathing and a bad cough. They may even need to be hospitalized. Doctors typically do give antibiotics for pneumonia. However, most children who have the flu but who don't have a bacterial infection at the same time don't need antibiotics. *Antiviral* medicines may be able to help children with the flu, however. Four antiviral medicines are available, although only two are useful for seasonal influenza: Tamiflu (oseltamivir) and Relenza (zanamivir). The other two medicines are no longer useful because influenza viruses have become resistant to them. Keep in mind these considerations about Tamiflu and Relenza:

- Children who are not very sick from the flu, or who don't have any other health problems that can make influenza worse (such as conditions of the lungs, heart, immune system, or nervous system), usually don't need antiviral medicines. These medications will not help much, if at all.

- Children who are very sick from influenza, especially children sick enough to be in a hospital, will more likely benefit from antiviral medicines.

- Children with other underlying health problems affecting the lungs, heart, immune system, nervous system, or other problems, such as diabetes, will more likely benefit from antiviral medicines.

- Younger children—under 2 years of age—are more likely to benefit from antiviral medicines.

- The antiviral medicines work best if given within 48 hours of when a child first starts to become sick. The antiviral medicines work by stopping the virus from reproducing and spreading, and, after 48 hours, much of the virus has already reproduced and spread in the body.

- The benefits of these antiviral medicines may be described as "modest." For many children who are otherwise healthy, they

will not help much, if at all; for some children, the medicines
may allow them to get better one or two days sooner than they
would if they had not received the medicine.

- The antiviral medicines can be expensive.

- Like any medicine, the antiviral medicines may cause side
effects (such as nausea and vomiting).

To return to the question at the beginning of this section, your
daughter's symptoms began three days ago, and even though she
feels bad from the flu, she doesn't need to be put in a hospital. Although the antiviral medicines may help some children recover faster from the flu, they need to be given soon after the illness begins—
preferably within 48 hours of when the child first begins to feel bad.
Because she has already been sick for 72 hours, antiviral medicines
probably will not help her much, if at all.

In our society, if a medicine is available for a specific illness, many
people believe that taking the medicine will make the illness go away
completely. For some medicines, this is not true. And just as bacteria
can become resistant to antibiotics, viruses can become resistant to
antiviral medicines. The more these medicines are used, the more
likely the viruses will become resistant. This is another important
reason why we like to use these medicines only when they are most
necessary; in other words, we like to use them wisely. These antiviral
medicines can be expensive, and like any medicine, they may cause
side effects (including nausea and vomiting).

There are, of course, some medicines you can give your daughter
to help her feel better. These include acetaminophen (Tylenol) or
ibuprofen (Motrin or Advil) for fever and discomfort. Nose sprays
with saline (salt solution) and humidifiers can aid a stuffy nose.
Nasal decongestant sprays may provide some comfort (but don't
give these for longer than five days). Cough medicines probably will
not make your daughter feel better. Try cough drops or hard candy.
Honey may help (though it should not be given to children younger
than 12 months old). Rest, a lot of fluids, and hot soup (try chicken
soup) also can help, just like your grandmother told you. Never give
aspirin to a child with the flu because aspirin may cause a potentially

deadly condition called Reye's syndrome when it is taken by a child who has the flu.

A virus causes the flu. Antibiotics are usually not necessary. Two antiviral medicines may help some children with the flu. Children who are not very sick or have been ill for a few days usually don't need these antiviral medicines. Children who are very sick from the flu, or who have certain health problems, may benefit from these antiviral medicines.

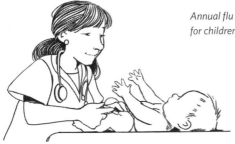

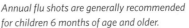
Annual flu shots are generally recommended for children 6 months of age and older.

My daughter is beginning to feel better after being sick with the flu for about a week. I don't want to go through that again! What can I do to prevent my other children from getting the flu?

The best way to protect you and your family from getting the flu is to be vaccinated with the flu vaccine. Influenza viruses change year to year, so it is important to receive a flu vaccine *every year*. Almost every year the flu vaccine differs, and it contains parts of the flu strains most likely to cause infection for that year.

While nearly anyone can benefit from receiving the flu vaccine, medical experts and the Centers for Disease Control and Prevention (CDC), the federal government agency that makes health-related recommendations for the public, say that specific people are most likely to benefit from the flu vaccine:

- all children 6 months of age and older (and especially children under 5 years of age);

- caregivers of infants less than 6 months of age, such as parents, grandparents, and child care workers (because infants less than 6 months of age can't be vaccinated, it's best to vaccinate those taking care of the infant); and

- certain adults.

Children younger than 5 years of age and children with certain underlying health problems are most likely to benefit from flu immunization because the flu can make these children very sick; it may even be deadly. These health problems include diabetes and medical conditions affecting the lungs (such as asthma), heart, immune system, and neuromuscular system. Children 8 years of age and younger who have not received a flu vaccine before should get two doses (one month apart) to help their immune system make antibodies against the flu virus.

There are two types of flu vaccine—the flu shot and the nose spray. The flu shot can be given to children 6 months of age and older while the nose spray is only given to children 2 years of age and older (because it was only studied in this age group). The flu shot is a mixture of parts of the flu virus; it does not contain any live viruses. The nose spray does contain live flu viruses and works somewhat better than the flu shot at preventing infection or serious infection. The flu shot is still very effective, however. Although the nose spray contains live flu viruses, these viruses have been weakened so they will not cause illness. Some children should not get the nose spray, such as children with asthma or lung problems, or children with diabetes. In the 2009 flu season, children should have had two separate flu vaccines—one against seasonal flu and one against H1N1 flu. For the 2010–11 flu season, the flu vaccine contained the H1N1 virus and the seasonal flu virus together. The 2011–12 flu vaccine is similar to the flu vaccine used in 2010–11 (the virus strains used in the vaccine are the same).

Some people say, "My children and I don't need a flu shot. We've never had the flu before." While it's wonderful that some people have not had the flu before, this doesn't mean that they won't get sick with influenza this year or next year. Remember that the influenza virus is constantly changing, so some years the flu virus may be especially bad and make a lot of people sick. We can't predict when a bad flu season will be.

Other people say, "I don't want a flu shot. I got one last year, and I still got the flu." This is certainly possible. Many believe that the flu vaccine should protect them 100 percent from getting sick with the flu. The flu vaccine may not be 100 percent protective, but this does not mean that it is not doing what it is supposed to. How well the flu vaccine works depends on how well it matches the actual flu viruses that are spreading and making people sick. When they make flu vaccines each year, medical experts guess what types or strains of flu virus are most likely to be seen in the upcoming flu season. Some years the vaccine and the natural flu virus match well, and other years they don't match as well. When the vaccine and natural viruses match well, flu vaccine can reduce the chance of getting the flu by 65 to 90 percent. Just as important, flu vaccine may also reduce how sick someone becomes if he or she catches the flu. So, if your child had a flu shot but still gets the flu, he or she may not be as sick as a child who didn't get the vaccine; the unvaccinated child might miss a week or more of school from the flu, or may even have to go to the hospital. When someone says, "*I still got the flu!*" it could even be that he or she actually had a bad cold or had a virus causing vomiting or diarrhea (a "stomach flu"), not influenza.

In addition to getting the flu vaccine, you can protect your children from the flu by using good personal hygiene, as described above. This includes washing your hands properly and often.

For more information about vaccines, see chapter 5.

✳

The best way to reduce the chance of getting the flu is to get a flu vaccine. Because the virus that causes the flu changes from year to year, a flu vaccine is needed every year. Flu vaccines will not give you the flu.

My 3-year-old son has a cough, a temperature of 99.5°F, and green snot coming from his nose. He seems to have a cold, and so do I. Does he need an antibiotic?

Colds, also known as upper respiratory tract infections (URI), are common in children. Children get more colds than adults, and young children average six to eight colds per year. With most colds occurring in the fall and winter, children can have a cold every month, so it may seem that they are nearly always sick! Why do children, and adults, have more colds in the winter? The cold outside temperatures don't directly lead to colds, as many parents believe (my mother certainly did). When it's cold outside, we spend more time inside, where we are generally closer to other people, and it's easier to pass cold germs (viruses) to others by sneezing and coughing.

More than 200 different viruses can cause the common cold. Because viruses cause colds, and not bacteria, antibiotics do not help. Parents often believe that their child needs an antibiotic if the child has a fever or thick, disgusting-looking snot coming from the nose. When cold viruses first get into the nose, they cause the nose to make clear mucus, and the child's nose "runs." This mucus actually helps to wash away the viruses. After a few days, the child's immune system "kicks in," and it begins to fight the virus with infection-fighting cells called white blood cells. The mucus from the nose then changes to thick white or yellow, then maybe to a greenish color. This is normal and does not at all mean that an antibiotic is needed.

The Centers for Disease Control and Prevention have a good saying about colds: "Snort, sniffle, sneeze, no antibiotics please."

Colds are self-limiting, which means that they eventually go away naturally. Colds go away within ten days or less. If your son's cold does not go away or get better within ten days, then call his doctor, as he may have another medical condition. Parents of young infants (3 months or younger) with a cold and a fever should always be in contact with the infant's doctor, as young infants can become much sicker more quickly.

Although children's colds don't need specific treatment, there are some medicines that claim to help children feel better. The products known as cough and cold medicines that are available over-the-counter usually are not that helpful, however. What this means is that there is no proof (that is, no good medical studies) to show that they are effective in relieving symptoms of the common cold in children. These medicines can actually be dangerous. This danger was publicized in the news in 2008 and 2009, as explained below.

If my son doesn't need an antibiotic, are there other medicines I can give him?

Yes, certainly. There are some medicines that you can give your son to help him feel better until the cold goes away. If your son has a mildly high temperature of 99.5°F, medically speaking, it is not a fever (100.5°F or higher). However, if your son is uncomfortable, then you can give him acetaminophen (Tylenol) or ibuprofen (Motrin or Advil). Cough and a stuffy nose are often the most bothersome symptoms of a cold for a child. It is especially important to reduce nasal congestion in younger infants, as young infants have more difficulty breathing through their mouths. Young infants with a congested nose have trouble eating and taking a bottle because they can't breathe and eat at the same time.

To help your son's congested nose, you can use saline solution, which is available in pharmacies as nose spray or drops. Put the saline solution into his nose, wait a few minutes, and then have him blow his nose or use a bulb aspirator and suck out the mucus. You can use a plain bulb aspirator, which is easy to use and inexpensive, or you can purchase a battery-powered nasal aspirator (Cleanoz nasal aspirator), which sells for about $30. After putting the saline into his nose, wait a few minutes before using the nasal aspirator because the salty water helps to pull out the mucus.

Use a cool mist humidifier or a cool mist vaporizer also. The moisture (humidity) released into the air from a humidifier will help loosen the mucus in the nose. It is important to clean humidifiers properly according to the package directions because an unclean humidifier can spread germs into the air.

For children older than 4 years with a congested nose, a parent can try giving them a decongestant medicine such as phenylephrine (nose sprays or drops, such as Little Noses or Neo-Synephrine). Don't give phenylephrine for more than three to five days because using it longer than this can make nasal congestion worse. Giving phenylephrine or other decongestants, such as pseudoephedrine, orally may also help. However, because it is given orally, the child may have more side effects, such as difficulty sleeping or feeling "hyper" (as an adult may feel after drinking too much coffee).

There are many cough and cold medicine products that you can buy to treat a cold, but you should not use them for your son. In 2008, the Food and Drug Administration (FDA) and the manufacturers of over-the-counter cough and cold products announced that these products should not be used in children younger than 4 years of age because there is no proof that they work and because they may be dangerous. There are many reports of young children dying from these medicines. Many of the deaths were due to parents accidentally giving too much of the medicine. This is easy to do for two reasons. First, the amount of the liquid medicine is hard to measure accurately. Second, because the medicines do not work well, it is tempting to keep giving more and more of them. The Food and Drug Administration is currently considering whether or not to recommend that cough and cold products not be used in children younger than 11 years.

A few medical studies have examined whether cough and cold products work in young children, and none of these studies have found that they work. You may wonder how can they be sold, and why are there so many of these products on the pharmacy shelves? It's a bit complicated, but the short answer is that because there is better evidence that cough and cold products may work in adults, the FDA assumed that they would work in children as well. They recommended children's dosages, although these dosage recommendations did not come from scientific studies.

Don't give your son any combination cough and cold products, such as Dimetapp, PediaCare, or other products with "multi-symptom" in their name, unless your doctor specifically recommends them. If your doctor does recommend a combination product, ask what specific medicines the product should contain, and then ask a pharmacist to help you choose a product at the pharmacy. A "combination" product is a product advertised to treat more than one symptom of the common cold, such as cough and fever and nasal congestion. These products are popular because it is easier to give just one medicine to treat a child's cold symptoms. A problem with these products is that parents may not be aware of all of the separate ingredients in them. Acetaminophen (Tylenol), for instance, is included in some combination cough and cold products. Not knowing this, parents may give a child more acetaminophen separately. This can be dangerous because too much acetaminophen can cause serious liver damage (see chapter 2). A medical study published in 2010 found that many children's liquid over-the-counter products, including cough and cold products, were confusing to use. Many contained directions that differed from the dosing devices that came with the product. Some products did not even have a dosing device.

Be sure you know what specific medicines are included in a product, and how these medicines are supposed to help, before you give any of that product to your son. Don't hesitate to speak with a pharmacist when you buy these products. That's what we are there for. We want parents to ask us questions about medicines so we can help parents safely care for their children.

Other products that you can buy in a pharmacy to help children with a cold are products that contain camphor, menthol, and eucalyptus oil. The product that you may be most familiar with that contains these medicines is Vicks VapoRub. You can often recognize it just by its smell. No medical study had scientifically tested such medicines in children with colds until a study was published in a medical journal in 2010. This study compared Vicks VapoRub to petrolatum (Vaseline) in children ages 2 to 11 years with colds, when put onto the child's chest at night before bedtime. It found that Vicks VapoRub was somewhat better than petrolatum, in that children who had Vicks VapoRub slept better and felt better. Be careful, however, if you use Vicks VapoRub or another product that has camphor in it. Camphor can be dangerous if it is swallowed, and even the smallest jar available in a pharmacy can kill a young child if he or she ingests it.

Cough may be a very bothersome symptom of a cold. Keep in mind, however, that Mother Nature is smart: there often is a good reason for the symptoms of an illness. As I explain in chapter 3, there is some scientific reason to believe that a fever is actually good for a child with an infection, as the higher body temperature may help kill the germs causing the infection. A cough may also be good for a child with an infection because it helps to clear out mucus from the nose, throat, and lungs.

Medical experts generally agree that it is not usually necessary to try to stop a cough unless the cough is so bad that the child is vomiting or can't sleep. Still, our society seems to want to treat any symptom with medicine, and there are plenty of cough medicines to buy in a pharmacy. Do these cough medicines work? No. The most common medicine contained in cough products is called dextromethorphan. Several medical studies of dextromethorphan in children found that it didn't help to relieve cough. In 1997 the American Academy of Pediatrics, the professional organization of pediatricians, recommended not using dextromethorphan or codeine in children, as there is no proof that they work, and they may cause many side effects. (Codeine cough products can be purchased over the counter in some states.)

Saying that cough products don't work for children may not make sense to some parents. They are commonly sold in pharmacies and advertised a lot. Why are they so widely available if they aren't effective? The explanation is somewhat complicated. Over the years, the FDA assumed that over-the-counter cough medicines worked in children as they may do in some adults. Because they were used a lot, the FDA allowed them to be sold. These medicines frequently combine dextromethorphan with an expectorant, such as guaifenesin. A common product containing this combination is Robitussin DM. An expectorant is supposed to loosen mucus and help someone feel and breathe better. However, guaifenesin doesn't work in children either (there are no good studies to show that it works). It's better to use a humidifier.

What *can* you use to help your son's cough? Often cough drops or plain hard candy will make him feel better. It may not be the medicine in the cough drops that helps but the feeling of sucking on the hard cough drop or candy that feels good and soothes the throat. Warm liquids, such as warm apple cider or warm lemonade, can also be soothing for older children. A study published in 2007 found that buckwheat honey (1/2 teaspoonful for younger children and 2 teaspoonsful for adolescents) was better than dextromethorphan for nighttime cough due to a cold in children 2 to 18 years of age. In this study buckwheat honey and dextromethorphan were compared to no treatment, and dextromethorphan was found to be no better than no treatment at all. Honey should not be given to infants less than 1 year of age, as it may cause infant botulism.

Some parents may wish to try alternative or natural treatments to treat their child's cold, including herbal medicines or vitamins. However, there is no scientific evidence from studies that herbal medicines (such as echinacea), minerals (such as zinc), or vitamins (such as vitamin C) substantially relieve the symptoms of the common cold in children.

---

*

Viruses cause colds, and antibiotics do not treat colds or help with cold symptoms. Many cough and cold products can be purchased over the counter, but they should not be given to children younger than 4 years of age, as they don't work and may cause dangerous side effects. They also may not work for children older than 4 years of age. Use acetaminophen or ibuprofen, nasal saline spray, and a humidifier, instead of over-the-counter cough and cold products. Honey or cough drops can help a cough in older children.

My 10-year-old daughter has a sore throat that is really bothering her. We have an appointment this afternoon with her doctor. What antibiotic should I request for her?

A sore throat, or pharyngitis, is common in children. Viruses cause most sore throats, so antibiotics are not helpful or necessary. However, bacteria can also cause sore throat. The most common bacteria to cause sore throat are called Group A streptococcus, or "strep" throat. How do we know if it is a virus or bacteria causing your daughter's sore throat? Some doctors believe that they can look at a child's throat and tell if a virus or bacteria is the cause. Often this isn't accurate, however. The best way is to use a quick test where a swab specimen is taken from the throat; within minutes, the doctor can determine if the strep throat bacteria are present. If the test is negative, it is still possible that the bacteria are present, and a back-up culture should be taken (this can take 48 to 72 hours for the results). If the test is positive, then the doctor will prescribe an antibiotic. The antibiotic generally used, because it is very effective, is penicillin. For younger children who can't swallow a penicillin tablet, amoxicillin liquid is usually used (penicillin liquid doesn't taste good). As with other antibiotics, it is important to finish all of the tablets or liquid, which should be taken for ten days for strep throat. Antibiotics are used to treat strep throat, to help the child feel better, and to prevent rheumatic fever and kidney inflammation. So, whenever your daughter complains of a sore throat and sees a doctor, be sure that the doctor takes a throat swab for a strep test to see if an antibiotic is necessary.

You can use the same over-the-counter medicines discussed above for treating colds to help your daughter feel better: acetaminophen or ibuprofen, warm liquids, and cough drops or hard candy.

*

Viruses often cause a sore throat in children, although bacteria may also be a cause. A quick throat swab test at the doctor's office can usually determine if bacteria are the cause. Antibiotics should only be given for a sore throat if bacteria are causing it.

CHAPTER 5

Are Vaccines Dangerous?
Will They Protect My Child?

Few topics in children's medical care cause more fears among parents and stir more discussion in the media than vaccines. I recall a mother who came to our pediatric pulmonary (lung) clinic for a new appointment for her 7-month-old son. I was in the clinic room when the doctor was asking the mother questions about her son's medical history. The doctor asked if her son's pediatric immunizations were up-to-date. No, replied the mother; he had not had any pediatric vaccines. (An infant normally would have had several injections of six vaccines throughout the first 6 months.) I asked the mother if she was concerned about side effects of vaccines, and if so, what side effects. She responded, "Yes. Death."

The medical profession considers childhood vaccines to be one of the ten greatest public health achievements of the past 100 years. Vaccines have saved millions of lives from infectious diseases such as polio, smallpox, and meningitis. How can there be such a wide difference of opinion about vaccines? Why are vaccines controversial?

I realize that the subject of childhood vaccines may be confusing to parents. There is a lot of information available about vaccines—on the Internet, in newspapers, on popular television talk shows, and in books written entirely about vaccines. Some of this information claims that vaccines can be dangerous to young infants. With so much conflicting information, who and what should you believe?

In this chapter I address questions about childhood vaccination:

- How do vaccines work? What are vaccines made of?
- Who decides what vaccines are recommended for my child?
- How effective are vaccines?
- What diseases do childhood vaccines protect against?
- What side effects do vaccines have? Are they dangerous?
- What concerns and fears do parents have about vaccines?
- What fears do children have about vaccines?
- Do vaccines have mercury in them? Is mercury dangerous? Do vaccines cause autism?
- Can I rely on other immunized children to protect my un-immunized child?
- What are good information sources about vaccines?
- What can I do if I have concerns about vaccines?

How do vaccines work? What are vaccines made of?

Our immune systems are amazing as they work to protect us from many types of germs—viruses, bacteria, and parasites—that exist in our world. Without an immune system, infants would not live long past birth. Immunization with a vaccine causes our immune systems to produce immunity—protection—against a specific infectious disease. Vaccines are the medicines we use for the process of immunization.

Children who receive a vaccine develop immunity against the viruses or bacteria contained in that vaccine. This immunity protects them from the disease that those viruses or bacteria cause. If immunized children are exposed to these germs (at school or from a friend, say), they will be much less likely to get the disease. And even if they do get the disease, it will be less severe and they will not be as sick. Our immune system remembers, from the vaccine, what a specific virus or bacteria looks like (chemically speaking, that is) and then attacks the germs if they get into the body. Think of the immune system as soldiers who can recognize and remember (from the vaccine) what the enemy (the virus or bacteria) looks like and quickly kill it.

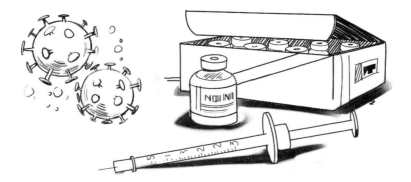

Vaccines help prevent diseases caused by viruses and bacteria.

Vaccines may contain parts of viruses or bacteria that cause disease, or they may contain the whole virus. When introduced into the body in a vaccine, these parts of the bacteria and viruses cause the person's immune system to make antibodies and other protective cells that then protect the person from the infections and diseases the bacteria and viruses cause. Some vaccines contain live viruses, but these live viruses have been attenuated (weakened). The immune system still produces protective antibodies against attenuated live vaccines. The MMR (measles, mumps, and rubella), varicella (chicken pox), rotavirus, and nasal influenza vaccines all contain live, weakened viruses. Most vaccines are made from inactivated viruses or bacteria, either as whole, killed viruses or as parts of viruses or bacteria.

Vaccines also contain fluid, and some include preservatives. The fluid in some vaccines, such as influenza vaccine, contains egg proteins from the manufacturing process. A child who has a severe allergy to eggs, one that causes difficulty breathing or throat swelling, should not have the influenza vaccine. Some vaccines used to include thimerosal as a preservative, but because of the concern some people had about thimerosal, which is chemically related to mercury, it was removed from nearly all vaccines. Thimerosal is now an ingredient in only a few types of influenza vaccine. There is more information about thimerosal later in this chapter.

Who decides what vaccines are recommended for my child?

Each year a schedule of the vaccines that are routinely recommended for infants, children, and adolescents is published, usually at the beginning of the year. These schedules are posted on the Centers for Disease Control and Prevention's (CDC) Web site (www.cdc.gov/vaccines) and other Web sites. The Advisory Committee on Immunization Practices of the CDC, the American Academy of Pediatrics, and the American Academy of Family Physicians work together to write the childhood and adolescent immunization schedules. These groups are composed of national experts (doctors and scientists) on infectious diseases and pediatrics. They review the latest information about vaccines and recent disease trends to determine what vaccines are best to prevent serious disease in infants, children, and adolescents. (For the infant and children schedules for 2012, see charts 5.1 and 5.2.)

Most vaccines are given in the first two years of an infant's life. Many parents wonder whether these vaccines could be spread out, an approach the author of one current vaccine book for parents has recommended. The timing and scheduling of the recommended childhood vaccinations is based on several important factors, including when (at what age) these germs are more likely to cause infection and disease and how an infant's immune system develops. Some infections are more likely to occur in younger infants than in older children. These vaccines should be given within an infant's first two years, as recommended in the immunization schedule. In addition, some of the vaccines must be given several times (in several doses) over several months to provide good protection against the disease-causing germs. So, it is best if the vaccines are given at the times recommended in the schedules in charts 5.1 and 5.2.

For various reasons, some parents may ask that some of their child's immunizations be given at different times or ages from what is recommended in the official pediatric immunization schedule. Some doctors are willing to give vaccines on a different schedule; others are not. I believe, as I explained above, that the pediatric immunizations should be given as listed in the schedule. Medical

experts have carefully evaluated administering the pediatric immunizations at the specific ages recommended in the schedules, and
your child will be protected most from dangerous infections if his or
her immunizations are given at these ages. If you have questions or
concerns about the immunization schedule, speak with your child's
doctor. The Web sites of the CDC and the American Academy of Pediatrics have additional information about vaccines for parents (www.
cdc.gov and www.aap.org).

How effective are vaccines?

Vaccines are very effective in preventing disease or reducing severity
of illness from disease. Like any medicine, however, vaccines are not
100 percent effective. As mentioned in chapter 4, some parents don't
want their child to get the flu shot this year because they had the shot
last year and still got the flu. While it is true that a child who had a flu
shot can still get the flu that year, it's likely that this child was much
less sick than if he had not had a flu shot.

The flu vaccine's effectiveness also varies from year to year. This
is because the flu viruses usually change each year, and to make
enough vaccine by September and October (which is when flu vaccines are usually first given for the upcoming flu season), experts
and pharmaceutical companies have to make an educated guess as
to what types of flu viruses will make us sick during the next flu season. Sometimes this guess is good, and sometimes it isn't as good.
The more closely the types of flu viruses in the vaccine match the flu
viruses causing disease during a flu season, the more effective the
vaccine will be. If the flu vaccine is not as effective one year, some
parents may lose faith in all flu vaccines, and they may not want their
child to have it the next year.

In past years, when the types of flu viruses in the vaccine closely
matched the flu types in the community, the flu vaccine has been 70
to 90 percent effective in preventing children from getting the flu.
During the 2003–2004 flu season, the types of flu viruses in the community did not closely match the types of viruses in the vaccine, and
the flu vaccine was 60 percent effective in preventing the flu. Even
when the match is not as similar, the flu vaccine may still help many

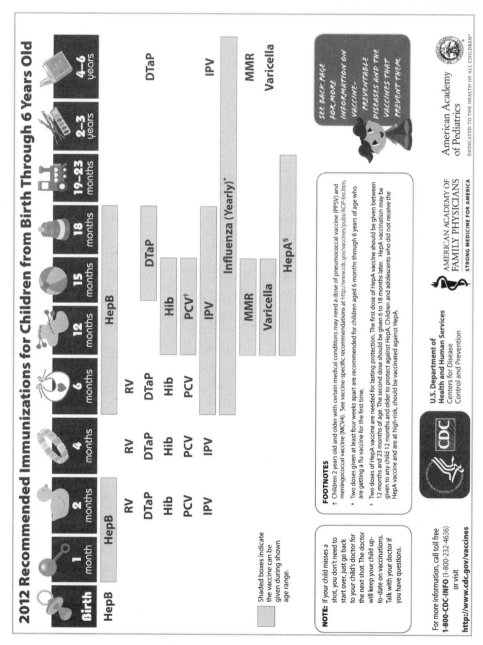

CHART 5.1
Recommended immunization schedule for persons aged 0 through 6 years—United States, 2012
Source: Courtesy of the Department of Health and Human Services, Centers for Disease Control and Prevention

---

2012 Recommended Immunizations for Children from Birth Through 6 Years Old

	Birth	1 month	2 months	4 months	6 months	12 months	15 months	18 months	19–23 months	2–3 years	4–6 years
HepB	HepB	HepB			HepB						
RV			RV	RV	RV						
DTaP			DTaP	DTaP	DTaP		DTaP				DTaP
Hib			Hib	Hib	Hib	Hib					
PCV			PCV	PCV	PCV	PCV†					
IPV			IPV	IPV	IPV						IPV
Influenza					Influenza (Yearly)*						
MMR						MMR					MMR
Varicella						Varicella					Varicella
HepA						HepA§					

Shaded boxes indicate the vaccine can be given during shown age range.

NOTE: If your child misses a shot, you don't need to start over, just go back to your child's doctor for the next shot. The doctor will keep your child up-to-date on vaccinations. Talk with your doctor if you have questions.

For more information, call toll free 1-800-CDC-INFO (1-800-232-4636) or visit
http://www.cdc.gov/vaccines

FOOTNOTES

† Children 2 years old and older with certain medical conditions may need a dose of pneumococcal vaccine (PPSV) and meningococcal vaccine (MCV4). See vaccine-specific recommendations at http://www.cdc.gov/vaccines/pubs/ACIP-list.htm.

* Two doses given at least four weeks apart are recommended for children aged 6 months through 8 years of age who are getting a flu vaccine for the first time.

§ Two doses of HepA vaccine are needed for lasting protection. The first dose of HepA vaccine should be given between 12 months and 23 months of age. The second dose should be given 6 to 18 months later. HepA vaccination may be given to any child 12 months and older to protect against HepA. Children and adolescents who did not receive the HepA vaccine and are at high-risk, should be vaccinated against HepA.

SEE BACK PAGE FOR MORE INFORMATION ON VACCINE-PREVENTABLE DISEASES AND THE VACCINES THAT PREVENT THEM.

U.S. Department of Health and Human Services
Centers for Disease Control and Prevention

AMERICAN ACADEMY OF FAMILY PHYSICIANS
STRONG MEDICINE FOR AMERICA

American Academy of Pediatrics
DEDICATED TO THE HEALTH OF ALL CHILDREN®

2012 Recommended Immunizations for Children from 7 Through 18 Years Old

7–10 YEARS	11–12 YEARS	13–18 YEARS
Tdap[1]	Tetanus, Diphtheria, Pertussis (Tdap) Vaccine	Tdap
	Human Papillomavirus (HPV) Vaccine (3 Doses)[2]	HPV
MCV4	Meningococcal Conjugate Vaccine (MCV4) Dose 1[3]	MCV4 Dose 1[3] — Booster at age 16 years
	Influenza (Yearly)[4]	
	Pneumococcal Vaccine[5]	
	Hepatitis A (HepA) Vaccine Series[6]	
	Hepatitis B (HepB) Vaccine Series	
	Inactivated Polio Vaccine (IPV) Series	
	Measles, Mumps, Rubella (MMR) Vaccine Series	
	Varicella Vaccine Series	

These shaded boxes indicate when the vaccine is recommended for all children unless your doctor tells you that your child cannot safely receive the vaccine.

These shaded boxes indicate the vaccine should be given if a child is catching-up on missed vaccines.

These shaded boxes indicate the vaccine is recommended for children with certain health conditions that put them at high risk for serious diseases. Note that healthy children **can** get the HepA series[6]. See vaccine-specific recommendations at www.cdc.gov/vaccines/pubs/ACIP-list.htm.

FOOTNOTES

[1] Tdap vaccine is combination vaccine that is recommended at age 11 or 12 to protect against tetanus, diphtheria and pertussis. If your child has not received any or all of the DTaP vaccine series, or if you don't know if your child has received these shots, your child needs a single dose of Tdap when they are 7–10 years old. Talk to your child's health care provider to find out if they need additional catch-up vaccines.

[2] All 11 or 12 year olds – both girls *and* boys – should receive 3 doses of HPV vaccine to protect against HPV-related disease. Either HPV vaccine (Cervarix® or Gardasil®) can be given to girls and young women; only one HPV vaccine (Gardasil®) can be given to boys and young men.

[3] Meningococcal conjugate vaccine (MCV) is recommended at age 11 or 12. A booster shot is recommended at age 16. Teens who received MCV for the first time at age 13 through 15 years will need a one-time booster dose between the ages of 16 and 18 years. If your teenager missed getting the vaccine altogether, ask their health care provider about getting it now, especially if your teenager is about to move into a college dorm or military barracks.

[4] Everyone 6 months of age and older—including preteens and teens—should get a flu vaccine every year. Children under the age of 9 years may require more than one dose. Talk to your child's health care provider to find out if they need more than one dose.

[5] A single dose of Pneumococcal Conjugate Vaccine (PCV13) is recommended for children who are 6 - 18 years old with certain medical conditions that place them at high risk. Talk to your healthcare provider about pneumococcal vaccine and what factors may place your child at high risk for pneumococcal disease.

[6] Hepatitis A vaccination is recommended for older children with certain medical conditions that place them at high risk. HepA vaccine is licensed, safe, and effective for all children of all ages. Even if your child is not at high risk, you may decide you want your child protected against HepA. Talk to your healthcare provider about HepA vaccine and what factors may place your child at high risk for HepA.

For more information, call toll free **1-800-CDC-INFO** (1-800-232-4636) or visit **http://www.cdc.gov/vaccines/teens**

U.S. Department of **Health and Human Services**
Centers for Disease Control and Prevention

CDC

American Academy of Pediatrics
DEDICATED TO THE HEALTH OF ALL CHILDREN®

AMERICAN ACADEMY OF FAMILY PHYSICIANS
STRONG MEDICINE FOR AMERICA

CHART 5.2
Recommended immunization schedule for persons aged 7 through 18 years—United States, 2011
Source: Courtesy of the Department of Health and Human Services, Centers for Disease Control and Prevention

children. The flu vaccine has other benefits. Studies have shown that the flu vaccine may reduce fever, doctor visits, use of antibiotics, and absence from school in children who still may catch the flu but not get as sick with the flu as they would have been without the vaccine.

Table 5.1 gives a snapshot of the effectiveness of childhood vaccines. It shows the decrease in the number of children who have had specific diseases from before vaccines were regularly used up to now. As you see, vaccines have been remarkably effective. These vaccines have been so effective that most of us alive today have never seen a child or adult with some of these diseases. If you had lived around 1920, you would probably have known several people who had polio or diphtheria or who even had died from one of these diseases. (In table 5.1, the number of children who had the disease before vaccines were used includes the years 1951 to 1954 for polio and 1920 to 1922 for diphtheria.)

We used to immunize against smallpox, but this disease has been eliminated from the world. The last naturally occurring case happened in 1977. Although the last case of polio in the United States was in 1979, the disease still occurs in some places (for example, in Africa), and it is still possible to get polio when traveling to these areas or when someone living in these countries travels to the United States (and brings the polio virus with them). So we continue to immunize against polio. All of the diseases that we currently immunize against (charts 5.1 and 5.2 and table 5.1) still occur in the United States (except polio), and although the number of children with these diseases has decreased because of vaccines, it is still possible for a child to become ill or even die from them. Therefore, children still need to receive vaccines against these diseases.

What diseases do childhood vaccines protect against?

The vaccines listed in chart 5.1 target 15 childhood diseases. As noted above, the viruses and bacteria that cause these diseases still exist in our communities (with the exception of the poliovirus), so it remains important for children to be immunized with these vaccines

TABLE 5.1 Incidence of several diseases, before and after vaccines (United States)

| | CHILDREN WITH DISEASE | | |
DISEASE	ANNUALLY (20TH CENTURY), PRIOR TO AVAILABILITY OF VACCINE	2007	% DECREASE
Diphtheria	175,885*	0	100.00
Pertussis (whooping cough)	147,271	10,454	93.00
Tetanus	1,314	28	98.00
Polio	16,316**	0	100.00
Measles	503,282	43	99.99
Mumps	152,209	800	99.50
Rubella (German measles)	47,745	12	99.99
Haemophilus influenzae type B (meningitis)	20,000	22	99.90

Source: American Academy of Pediatrics, *Red Book* (2009)
* 1920–22, ** 1951–54

to prevent illness and even death. Table 5.2 sets out what diseases these viruses and bacteria cause and what can happen if your child becomes ill from them.

> ✱ All of the diseases that childhood vaccines protect against can cause children to be very sick, and most of these diseases can kill children. Childhood vaccines can very effectively prevent these diseases, and they can reduce how sick children become if they do get the disease.

TABLE 5.2   Childhood diseases that vaccines protect against.

DISEASE	HOW IS THE DISEASE SPREAD?	WHAT TYPE OF ILLNESS CAN THE DISEASE CAUSE?	IS DEATH POSSIBLE FROM THIS DISEASE?
Hepatitis B virus	Birth from an infected mother; sex (adolescents); blood from an infected person; intravenous drug use	Hepatitis (liver disease)	Yes
Rotavirus	Contact with stool from an infected person	Diarrhea and dehydration	Yes
Diphtheria bacteria	Respiratory (coughing; sneezing; contact with nose, mouth)	Fever; sore throat; difficulty breathing	Yes
Tetanus (lockjaw) bacteria	Found in the soil and dirty areas and infects an open wound	Lockjaw; severe muscle spasms	Yes
Pertussis (whooping cough) bacteria	Respiratory (coughing; sneezing; contact with nose, mouth)	Cough; pneumonia	Yes
Haemophilus influenzae type B bacteria	Respiratory (coughing; sneezing; contact with nose, mouth)	Meningitis; pneumonia	Yes
Pneumococcal bacteria	Respiratory (coughing; sneezing; contact with nose, mouth)	Meningitis; pneumonia; ear infections	Yes
Poliovirus	Contact with stool from an infected person	Muscle paralysis	Yes
Influenza (flu) virus	Respiratory (coughing; sneezing; contact with nose, mouth)	Fever; cough; ear infections; muscle aches; headache; vomiting; pneumonia	Yes
Measles virus	Respiratory (coughing; sneezing; contact with nose, mouth)	Fever; cough; rash; pneumonia	Yes
Mumps virus	Respiratory (coughing; sneezing; contact with nose, mouth)	Swelling of salivary glands; fever; muscle aches	Yes, but rare and mostly in adults

TABLE 5.2 (continued)

DISEASE	HOW IS THE DISEASE SPREAD?	WHAT TYPE OF ILLNESS CAN THE DISEASE CAUSE?	IS DEATH POSSIBLE FROM THIS DISEASE?
Rubella (German measles) virus	Respiratory (coughing; sneezing; contact with nose, mouth)	Fever; rash—usually mild in children, but causes many birth defects if mother develops disease while pregnant	Most dangerous to a fetus (before birth)
Varicella (chicken pox) virus	Respiratory (coughing; sneezing; contact with nose, mouth)	Rash; skin infections; pneumonia; swelling of the brain	Yes
Hepatitis A virus	Contact with stool from an infected person	Fever; nausea; tiredness; jaundice	Yes
Meningococcal bacteria	Respiratory (coughing; sneezing; contact with nose, mouth)	Meningitis; severe whole body infection	Yes

What side effects do vaccines have? Are vaccines dangerous?

Like other medicines, vaccines are not 100 percent safe, and they may cause side effects. Side effects common to any vaccine injection (shot) are swelling, redness, and pain at the site of injection, fever, and rash. Some vaccines may cause more serious side effects. These side effects may include anaphylaxis (a severe allergic reaction that may cause difficulty breathing), arthritis-like joint pain, shoulder muscle weakness (brachial neuritis), seizure-like movements, or prolonged crying. Seizure-like movements that may result from a vaccine are caused by a high fever (105° or higher) and are not epilepsy. These side effects, although serious, rarely occur. For example, seizure-like movements may occur after the MMR vaccine in about 1 out of 3,000 shots, and anaphylaxis may occur in 1 out of 250,000. An older vaccine for diphtheria, tetanus, and pertussis (DTP) that is no longer given to infants used to cause more side effects than the currently used vaccine, DTaP. Seizure-like movements (caused by high fever) had occurred in about 1 out of 1,750 DTP shots. This side effect occurs far less often with the currently used DTaP vaccine—about 1 out of 14,000 shots. Some side effects, such as long-term seizures, deafness, or permanent brain damage, have been reported to occur so rarely after vaccines (1 out of 1,000,000 shots) that it is hard to determine accurately if the vaccine actually caused the side effect. I mention this here as you may find this information when reading about vaccines on various Web sites.

Another consideration that "muddies the waters" about vaccines and side effects is that some childhood medical conditions begin to occur at about the same time that vaccines are given—in the first one or two years of life. Some types of seizure disorders may first appear during this time. So if an infant or young child has a vaccine shot and a few days later he or she has a seizure, it's easy to blame the vaccine as the cause. Probably the best example of this coincidental timing is autism. Many types of autism exist, and the timing of when symptoms of autism first occur varies. Symptoms of autism often appear in the first several years of life, when many of the childhood vaccines are given. Because we don't yet know what causes autism, many parents have blamed vaccines (primarily the MMR vaccine) as the cause.

The risk of encephalopathy (swelling of the brain) as a serious side effect of the measles vaccine is 1 out of 1,000,000. However, the risk of encephalopathy from the disease measles is 1 out of 1,000. So the risk of brain swelling from the disease is one thousand times greater than from the vaccine.

Vaccines, like other medicines, have contraindications. A contraindication means that some infants or children with certain medical conditions should not receive a specific vaccine. If a child with a contraindication to a specific vaccine accidentally receives that vaccine, side effects are more likely to occur, and they may occur more severely. For example, giving a flu shot (which contains egg proteins from the manufacturing process) to a child with a severe egg allergy may cause serious side effects. Another example is children whose immune system is abnormal (from a disease or from chemotherapy for childhood cancer). If a family member living with a child is receiving chemotherapy for cancer, this may also be a reason for not giving certain immunizations to the child. These children should not receive the live-viral vaccines such as varicella (chicken pox), as it is possible for the attenuated virus to cause serious infection in a child with an abnormal immune system or in a person receiving chemotherapy (from the child "shedding" live virus). Before your child receives vaccines, the doctor should ask you questions to determine if your child or family members have any contraindications for vaccines. If your doctor doesn't ask, you should initiate the conversation with your doctor.

How is vaccine safety tested?

Pharmaceutical companies test vaccines, like other medicines, for ten years or more in several different phases before the Food and Drug Administration (FDA) allows them to be used in the general public. When a vaccine is approved for use for the public, the FDA has determined that the benefits of the vaccine (preventing or reducing disease) are greater than any of its risks (side effects), and that the vaccine is safe to use. After the FDA approves a vaccine and it is being used in many thousands of children, monitoring for safety does not stop. Safety monitoring, especially for rarer side effects, is done in several ways. Doctors and other health care professionals are asked to report side effects from vaccines when they see them, through a system called VAERS (Vaccine Adverse Event Reporting System). Other vaccine safety monitoring programs in place include the Vaccine Safety Datalink Project and the Clinical Immunization Safety Assessment Network.

A good example of the benefit of these safety-monitoring programs is an older vaccine named RotaShield. RotaShield was used in young infants to prevent diarrhea and dehydration from rotavirus. Reports to the Vaccine Adverse Event Reporting System in 1999 showed that RotaShield caused a rare but serious side effect called intussusception (where part of the intestinal tract folds over itself and becomes blocked, like a pair of socks folded in on each other). This side effect occurred in 1 of 10,000 children. RotaShield was discontinued, and a safer rotavirus vaccine is now used.

How do we measure risk versus benefit for vaccines?

As I discuss in chapter 1, the benefit and the risk of any medicine must be considered before it is used. For vaccines, this concept is of great importance. I believe that some parents don't adequately think about the benefits of vaccines when they decide not to immunize their children. Or perhaps they think too much about the risks of vaccines rather than the benefits. Many vaccines, such as polio or measles/mumps/rubella (MMR), have been so successful and effective in eliminating or reducing disease that it's easy to forget about these diseases. After all, when was the last time you heard of a child with polio? Some young pediatricians I know and work with have never seen a child with meningitis from the bacterial germ *Haemophilus influenzae* type B, which we now have a vaccine to protect against. When I first started working as a pediatric pharmacist, this germ caused many cases of meningitis. Meningitis is a horrible infection—if it doesn't kill the infant or child, it can cause him or her to be deaf or to have permanent brain damage. Now, meningitis due to this germ occurs very rarely, and when it does occur, it often is in an infant who did not receive this vaccine.

Some parents may believe that because the infectious diseases that we have vaccines for occur so rarely, these infections are no longer important, and their child no longer needs the vaccines. This is not true. All of the germs and diseases listed in table 5.2 are still present in our communities, except polio. (As mentioned above, the polio virus still exists in other countries, and it can travel with people who have been to these countries.) Consider this information from the Centers for Disease Control and Prevention:

- In 2004, 25,827 cases of pertussis (whooping cough) were reported in the United States.

- From 1989 to 1991, 55,000 cases of measles occurred in the United States, causing 132 deaths. Most of these deaths were in children.

- From 1988 to 1995 (before the chicken pox vaccine was available), 10,000 people were sick enough from chicken pox that they needed to be hospitalized. From 1990 to 1994, more than 40 children died each year from chicken pox—a total of more than 200 children.

- In 2008, five infants in Minnesota developed serious infection from the bacterial germ *Haemophilus influenzae* type B. One of the infants died. Three infants had not had any of the vaccines for this germ, and another had had only two vaccine doses (of a total of four doses normally given). The other infant had an abnormal immune system and thus was at a higher risk for infection.

- Children who do not receive the pertussis vaccine are 23 times more likely to get pertussis than children who do receive the vaccine.

I suggest that you think about childhood vaccines this way:

- Vaccines provide very good protection from dangerous infectious diseases. These diseases still occur in our communities, and they can make your child very sick. And nearly all of them can even kill your child.

- Yes, vaccines have side effects. But most of these side effects are not serious. Serious side effects may occur, but they occur very rarely.

- The risk of serious illness or death from infectious diseases is much greater than the small risk of serious side effects from vaccines.

- For most infants and children, the benefit of vaccines outweighs their risks. Some children with specific medical conditions should not receive some vaccines, however.

✱ Like any medicine, vaccines are not 100 percent safe. Vaccines do have side effects, although they are mostly minor, such as discomfort from a shot. More serious effects occur rarely. The benefits that vaccines offer in protecting children from dangerous infectious diseases are many times greater than the risk of serious side effects.

What concerns and fears do parents have about vaccines?

To find out more about what concerns and fears parents have about vaccines, researchers have conducted several surveys of parents. A leading pediatric medical journal published the results of one survey in 2010. Of the 1,552 parents surveyed, 90 percent believed that vaccines protect their child from disease. But these parents had worries about vaccines: 54 percent were concerned about serious side effects of vaccines; 25 percent believed that some vaccines caused autism in healthy children; and 12 percent had refused at least one vaccine recommended by their child's doctor. Many parents in this survey believed that their child was at a low risk of getting some of the diseases that vaccines target. Another study of more than 8,000 parents found that the percentage of those who refused or delayed vaccines for their child increased from 22 to 39 percent between 2003 and 2008. A major reason for this increase was because of concerns

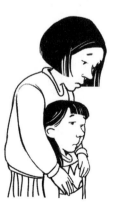

Many parents are concerned about the potential side effects of vaccines, but most parents understand that vaccines keep their child safe from serious infections.

TABLE 5.3 Beliefs and concerns parents may have about vaccines

BELIEF	SCIENTIFIC INFORMATION
Natural immunity is better than vaccines.	"Natural immunity" derives from a child having the disease; it involves a high risk of severe illness or death from the disease. Vaccines provide similar immunity with less risk.
Giving many vaccines at one time can "overload" a child's immune system.	The recommended vaccines given by the immunization schedule use only a small part of the immune system's ability to recognize and remember germs.
Vaccines can weaken a child's immune system.	If this were true, then children who have received vaccines would be at greater risk of disease, which is not the case.

Source: American Academy of Pediatrics, *Red Book* (2009)

about side effects of vaccines. If you have similar concerns about vaccines, then you are not alone. Table 5.3 lists several beliefs about vaccines that parents may have, along with the scientific perspective on these beliefs.

What fears do children have about vaccines?

I doubt that your child is worried about autism when he or she gets a vaccine. Instead, your child is fearful of the pain of a shot. This is the most common fear children have when they go to see their doctor: *"Am I going to get a shot?"* As I discussed in chapter 1, there are several methods you can use to help comfort your child when he or she gets a shot at the doctor's office. These methods may help to comfort your child—and you—when vaccines are given. (See chapter 1 for more information.)

Do vaccines cause autism? Do vaccines have mercury in them? Is mercury in vaccines dangerous?

Autism is probably the single biggest concern and fear that parents have about childhood vaccines. The topic of vaccines causing autism has been widely discussed in newspapers and books and on television, including popular programs such as the Oprah Winfrey Show.

TABLE 5.4   Internet sites with reliable vaccine information

SITE	AUTHORS AND ORGANIZATION
www.cdc.gov/vaccines	Centers for Disease Control and Prevention
www.aap.org/healthtopics/immunizations.cfm	American Academy of Pediatrics
www.kidsmeds.info	Pediatric Pharmacy Advocacy Group
www.familydoctor.org	American Academy of Family Physicians
www.vaccinesafety.edu	Institute for Vaccine Safety, Johns Hopkins University
www.pkids.org	Parents of Kids with Infectious Diseases
www.vaccine.chop.edu	Vaccine Education Center at the Children's Hospital of Philadelphia
www.immunizationinfo.org	National Network for Immunization Information
www.hmhb.org	National Healthy Mothers, Healthy Babies Coalition

Several celebrities, including Jenny McCarthy and Jim Carrey, have talked about how dangerous they believe vaccines to be, and their fame has gotten their beliefs a lot of attention.

The nation's experts in pediatric medicine, infectious diseases, and other sciences have officially stated that there is no scientific proof that vaccines or thimerosal (a mercury-based preservative that used to be in many vaccines) cause autism. The Internet sites listed in table 5.4 have information from these experts about this topic.

Autism, also known as autism spectrum disorders, affects a child's ability to communicate and interact with other people. It is a difficult disease for a family because it creates a distance between the child and the family, and it may cause a child to have difficult behaviors. We don't know exactly what causes autism, and that lack of understanding allows some people to blame vaccines as the cause.

Concern about a connection between autism and vaccines took off in 1998 with the publication of a paper in the British medical journal the *Lancet* about 12 children with autism or similar medical disorders. The paper's author, Dr. Andrew Wakefield, implied that the

MMR vaccine caused or contributed to the development of autism in these children. Soon after this paper was published, use of the MMR vaccine in the United Kingdom decreased from 95 percent to 50 percent, and rates of measles and rubella increased. Some children in the United Kingdom died from measles in this period, even though fatal measles in children had not occurred for many years prior to 1998. Reproducing a medical study's results by other scientists is a good way to prove any study's accuracy and reliability. So other scientists tried to reproduce Dr. Wakefield's study. These later studies had different results—they found that the MMR vaccine did not contribute to autism. Other, different studies compared the rates of autism in large groups of children who had and had not received the MMR vaccine. One of these studies compared over 500,000 children in Denmark and found no differences in the rate of autism in children who did not receive the MMR vaccine as compared to children who did receive it.

Since 1998, several studies have been published in medical journals, and all of them have found that the MMR vaccine does not cause, or contribute to, autism. In 2004, 10 of the 12 co-authors on Dr. Wakefield's study retracted their names and interpretation of this study; they stated that they no longer wanted their names linked to it. In 2010, the *Lancet* officially retracted the study. The journal's editors stated that the study was poorly done and that they were "taking the paper back," in part because Dr. Wakefield had broken several scientific rules for conducting a medical study of children. Also in 2010, the regulatory agency that licenses doctors in England, the General Medical Council, found Dr. Wakefield guilty of professional misconduct. The agency took away his medical license and banned him from practicing medicine in England. In early 2011, the *British Medical Journal* published reports further demonstrating that Dr. Wakefield's original 1998 study was conducted with major scientific errors and use of false data (information). Unfortunately, many people continue to believe that Dr. Wakefield's 1998 study was valid and that the MMR vaccine causes autism.

Because of all of the debate and concern about MMR vaccine and autism, and because many parents were refusing to have their children receive the MMR vaccine, the Institute of Medicine reviewed the studies on MMR and a possible link to autism. The Institute of Medicine is an independent, nonprofit organization of scientists and experts that works outside of the government to provide unbiased recommendations and advice to the public and medical professionals. In 2004, it concluded that "*the body of epidemiologic evidence favors rejection of a causal relationship between the MMR vaccine and autism.*" *Epidemiologic evidence* refers to studying patterns and contributing factors about health and illness in large groups or populations of people. In other words, these experts said that there is no evidence that the MMR vaccine causes autism.

Another concern that some have raised about the dangers of childhood vaccines is the use of a preservative called thimerosal, once found in many vaccines. Thimerosal, which was first used in the 1950s, contains *ethyl* mercury, and mercury can be dangerous to our nervous systems and the brain. Some have claimed that thimerosal has contributed to autism. This topic can be confusing because much of what we know about the dangers of mercury comes from studying *methyl* mercury, which is found in the environment as an organic form of mercury. But *ethyl* mercury (as thimerosal) is chemically different from *methyl* mercury, and they work differently in our bodies. In addition, the amount of ethyl mercury (as thimerosal) that had been included in vaccines was very small. Even though there are chemical differences between these types of mercury, thimerosal was taken out of most childhood vaccines by 2001. Thimerosal was never proven to be dangerous, but the pharmaceutical companies removed it, out of fears of potential lawsuits and to prevent parents from refusing to use vaccines for their children. Other than some flu vaccines, none of the recommended childhood vaccines in chart 5.1 currently contain thimerosal.

If thimerosal does cause autism, we might expect to find that autism rates had decreased after the removal of thimerosal from vaccines. This has not happened; in fact, rates of autism have actually increased since 2001. There is much information that shows that thimerosal does not cause autism. One body of evidence comes from Iraq in 1971, when wheat used to make bread was contaminated with *methyl* mercury. Many people in Iraq ate the contaminated bread, resulting in one of the largest single-source mercury intoxications ever recorded. A total of 6,500 people were hospitalized, and 450 people died. Pregnant women who ate this bread gave birth to infants with many nervous system conditions, but an increase in autism did not occur. Several large studies have compared rates in autism between thousands of children who received thimerosal-containing vaccines and children who received vaccines without thimerosal in the United States and other countries. None of these studies have shown that children who had vaccines with thimerosal were more likely to develop autism. Also, the Institute of Medicine has reviewed all the studies and scientific information about thimerosal and has concluded that *"the body of epidemiological evidence favors rejection of a causal relationship between thimerosal-containing vaccines and autism."*

The Internet sites listed in table 5.4 include links to the full reports by the Institute of Medicine, which contain additional information about the scientific evidence concerning vaccines, thimerosal, and autism.

> ✳
> Vaccines and thimerosal (a mercury-based preservative) do not cause autism. Many scientific studies have shown this. Most vaccines no longer contain thimerosal. Not giving vaccines to your child because of concerns about vaccines causing autism increases the risk of your child getting, and dying from, dangerous infectious diseases.

Can I rely on other immunized children to protect my un-immunized child?

Some parents are comforted by the belief that even if their child is not immunized, other children who have been immunized will protect their child. This is called "herd immunity." To some extent, the principle behind such a belief is true. Other children who have been immunized will protect a child who has not been immunized. However, as I discussed above, the germs that vaccines protect against still exist in our communities and environment. So, an unvaccinated child who comes in contact with these germs remains much more susceptible to the diseases they cause. Also, the more children who are not immunized, the higher the chances are that the diseases may be spread from child to child.

Relying on "herd immunity" to protect your child may be dangerous to other children. As discussed above, there are some infants or children who shouldn't receive vaccines because of their young age or because they have other medical conditions that prevent them from receiving vaccines. These children are more susceptible to infectious diseases, and one of the best ways to protect them is to surround them with others who have been immunized. For example, an infant younger than 6 months is too young to receive a flu shot, but influenza (the flu) may be dangerous to these young infants. One of the best ways to protect these young infants is for others near them (siblings, parents, grandparents) to be immunized. The same is true for an infant or young child born with an abnormal immune system or a child with childhood cancer (such as leukemia) who is being treated with chemotherapy (because chemotherapy weakens the immune system as part of the treatment for cancer). Infections like chicken pox may be especially dangerous to these children, and unvaccinated children can pass these germs along to susceptible children more easily.

What are good sources of information about vaccines?

With so much conflicting information available, it is easy to understand how parents may become confused about vaccines. Simply typing "childhood vaccines" into an Internet search engine results in hundreds of sites. Many of these sites state that while childhood vaccines may have some side effects, they are safe and effectively protect children from infectious diseases. Other sites describe how terrible childhood vaccines are and how they are "poisoning" our children. Whom should you believe?

Table 5.4 lists several Internet sites that I believe you can trust to provide factually correct information. The first two sites listed in this table are good places to start. They are from the Centers for Disease

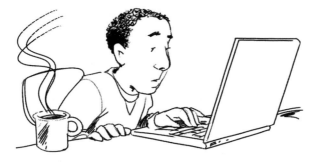

Control and Prevention and the American Academy of Pediatrics. Our country's best experts in pediatric medicine and infectious diseases review the information about vaccines on these sites. These sites are written specifically for parents in nonmedical language and are easy to understand. Keep in mind that anyone can set up a Web site and write anything he or she wants about vaccines. If the Web site *looks* professional, it becomes easier to believe the information there. (See chapter 7 for more information about how to rate the quality of an Internet site.)

These books about childhood vaccines are also reliable sources of information:

Autism's False Prophets: Bad Science, Risky Medicine, and the Search for a Cure, by Dr. Paul Offit. Dr. Offit is a pediatric infectious diseases doctor at the Children's Hospital of Philadelphia. This book is an interesting and informative discussion of the claim that many have made about vaccines causing autism. Dr. Offit describes how misleading and dangerous these claims have been.

Do Vaccines Cause That?! A Guide for Evaluating Vaccine Safety Concerns, by Martin Myers and Diego Pineda. This book is a very good resource for parents who have questions or concerns about vaccine safety.

Factcines: Facts on Vaccines, Just the Data. You Decide, by Dr. Susan Shoshana Weisberg. Dr. Weisberg is a pediatrician in Highland Park, Illinois. Her writing is easy to understand.

What can I do if I still have concerns about vaccines?

I hope this chapter has helped answer most, if not all, of your questions and concerns about vaccines. But if you continue to worry about vaccines, what can you do? One of the best ways to address your concerns is to write them down and discuss them with your child's doctor. Share your questions with your child's doctor, being open and specific about your concerns. Also, take some time to look at the Internet sites listed in table 5.4. These Web sites will address many of the questions you have, particularly about vaccines and autism, serious side effects of vaccines, and giving many vaccines simultaneously.

✱

> There is a lot of information available about vaccines, but much of it is not scientifically accurate. Use reputable Internet sites to read more about vaccines. Talk to your child's doctor if you have concerns or questions about vaccines and the diseases they protect against.

What vaccines do you—the author—and your family get?

Because I believe that vaccines are a very effective means to protect myself and my family from dangerous infectious diseases, I personally have had all of the vaccines that are recommended for adults. Each year I get a flu shot. I have never had influenza, and I would like to keep it that way. I don't want to be sick in bed for days. My wife also gets a flu shot each year. And my two children, now teenagers, have had all of the childhood vaccines recommended by the American Academy of Pediatrics, including flu vaccines each year.

CHAPTER 6

How Do I Use Medicines for Common Illnesses?

Common childhood medical conditions include head lice, diarrhea, constipation, pain, asthma, and attention-deficit hyperactivity disorder (ADHD). Some of these common childhood ailments can be treated with over-the-counter medicines, which you can purchase in a pharmacy without a doctor's prescription. Other medicines require a prescription. In this chapter I talk about how well these medicines work, their side effects, and the differences between the many medicines that can be used for the same illness. Common childhood infections, such as the common cold, ear infections, and the flu, and the medicines for treating them, are discussed in chapter 4.

Questions that you may have about medicines used for common childhood conditions include:

- Do over-the-counter medicines for head lice really work? Are they safe?
- Which medicine is better for treating my child's pain— Tylenol or Motrin?
- Can I use antidiarrheal medicine for my child when he has diarrhea?
- Are steroid medicines safe for my child with asthma?
- Are Ritalin and other medicines for attention-deficit hyperactivity disorder (ADHD) addicting?

HEAD LICE

Only children from dirty homes have head lice, right?

Infections with head lice are very common in children. Most head lice infections occur when school begins; the children are close together, and head lice can easily pass from one child to another. Here are some common misconceptions about head lice:

- "A child with head lice comes from a dirty home." *Not true.* Having head lice has nothing to do with being dirty or living in a dirty home. Even a child who lives in a mansion and wears expensive new clothes can have head lice. Any child can have head lice, if he or she is exposed to another child with head lice.

- "Head lice can jump from one child to another child." *Not true.* Head lice do not jump or fly. They are small (about the size of a sesame seed), and they can move quite fast, but they do not jump. They pass from one child to another by direct contact, such as when children hug (their hair touches) or goof around or wrestle on the floor. Head lice can also pass from one child to another when sharing clothes (such as hats) or personal items (such as combs or hairbrushes), although this is not as likely.

- "Head lice can pass dangerous diseases." *Not true.* Head lice do not pass any diseases, and they are not dangerous. Some children may not even know they have head lice, although head lice may cause itching. The main reason to treat head lice is the unpleasant thought of having small critters crawling in your hair and the social stigma of having head lice (not because they are dangerous). Certainly, if a child is known to have head lice, other children will make fun and not want to be near the child. Schools will not allow children to be in class if they have head lice.

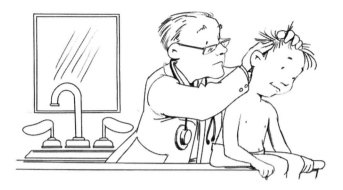

I have heard that many children in my child's school have head lice. How do I know if my child has head lice?

The best way to find out whether your child has head lice is to have your child's doctor look through your child's hair. Doctors diagnose head lice by seeing the head lice in the hair. You may try to find them, but head lice are small and can move fast. The best place to see head lice is the back of your child's head, near the neckline, or in the hair behind the ears. It's easy to be fooled, however, as small particles (such as dandruff) can look like lice. One medical study found that about half of all "head lice" sent to researchers by teachers and doctors (who thought they were sending head lice samples) were actually skin particles, dandruff, and other things. Doctors will often use a large magnifying glass when looking through a child's hair to help find lice.

Yuck! The doctor says my child does have head lice! Do over-the-counter head lice medicines work? Are they safe?

Many, but not all, of the medicines for head lice that you can buy in a pharmacy without a doctor's prescription can effectively kill your child's head lice. These medicines are inexpensive, and some do work well. The American Academy of Pediatrics 2010 guidelines on treating head lice recommend first trying over-the-counter medicine. The most common over-the-counter brands are Nix (permethrin),

RID (pyrethrin), and A-200 (pyrethrin). All of these also come as generic products, which are usually less expensive. I believe that the generic products work just as well as the more expensive trade-name products.

Other than these permethrin or pyrethrin products, I do not recommend using lice products you may see on the pharmacy shelf. There is not enough evidence that the other products work. Chances are good that the permethrin and pyrethrin products will kill all of the lice and eggs that your child has. However (and this is a big however), it is important that you use the product correctly. This means using it *exactly* as the directions on the label instruct. Different products have different directions, so be sure to read the bottle carefully. For example, do not use Nix just after shampooing with a combination shampoo and creme rinse product or a separate creme rinse. Creme rinses coat the hair, so the medicine doesn't work as well. Different products must be left on hair for different lengths of time, whether applying to wet or dry hair.

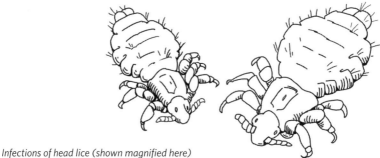

Infections of head lice (shown magnified here)
are easily spread among children.

All of the products must be used again in 7 to 10 days after first use, to kill any eggs that hatched in the meantime. Your child's doctor may tell you to reapply the product twice, once at day 7, 8, or 9 and again on day 13, 14, or 15. If you forget to do this, the eggs will hatch, and your child will have head lice again! If you used one of these products correctly and it didn't kill the head lice, it's possible that the lice are resistant to the medicine. In the past few years, resistance has become a big concern of doctors. If your child's head lice are resistant, then you will need to use a prescription medicine.

The head lice medicines you can buy over the counter are safe. They have been used for many years, and there are no reports of serious side effects from using them. They may cause some mild redness or itching on your child's scalp, but this is not likely to be serious. You may read on some Internet sites that these products are dangerous. Some people believe that chemical head lice medicines should not be used on young children because they are "insecticides." These products are chemicals (as are all medications), but there are no reports of dangerous side effects when they are used properly.

Some parents do not want to use chemical medicines on their child. There are "natural" products that you can buy, but there is not as much scientific evidence that they work well. Scientific evidence is evidence from scientific studies, not word-of-mouth evidence (such as "I've tried them in my children and they work"). Also, these natural products are not regulated by the Food and Drug Administration as over-the-counter products are. This means that their purity (how much active ingredient is in the product) may not be accurately reflected by what is listed on the package label. It also means that their safety is not as well regulated. If you do want to try a natural product, you can try Hair-Clean 1-2-3. This product may work as well as permethrin products (such as Nix). I would not recommend using products that try to suffocate lice, such as Vaseline, mayonnaise, or olive oil, as there is no evidence that they work, and what a mess they make. You'll spend many hours trying to clean this stuff out of your child's hair.

I tried an over-the-counter head lice medicine, and it didn't work. Will prescription products work better?

Yes, it is likely that a prescription product will work better to kill your child's head lice. The downside is that you will need to bring your child to the doctor, and the prescription products are likely to be more expensive. There are several effective prescription products. I believe the medicine that is most effective is Ovide (malathion). However, this medicine can be expensive—more than $100 if you have no insurance. Ovide has a lot of isopropyl alcohol in it, which means that it can catch fire easily, and because of this, it can be very dangerous to use. It is important to use Ovide exactly as you are told and not to apply it to your child's head near a heat source (including a hair dryer). After applying Ovide, and while your child's hair is still wet, don't use an iron or curling iron near your child. Other than this concern, Ovide is safe to use, and its side effects are usually minor, such as mild scalp irritation. Other prescription products that may also work include Ulesfia (benzyl alcohol), Natroba (spinosad), or ivermectin. (Ivermectin should not be used on younger children less than about 30 pounds.) These medicines are generally safe to use and may cause only minor side effects, none of them known to be serious.

My child's head lice are gone, finally!
What can I do to prevent this from happening again?

If you have more than one child, you should check (and probably treat) your other children (and anyone else who lives in your home) for head lice. It is easy for a child to become reinfected with head lice from someone else. Although it is not likely that your child got head lice from another child's hat or comb, it is still possible. So tell your child not to share hats, combs, hairbrushes, or clothes with others. Only things that touched your child's head in the 24 to 48 hours before treatment need to be cleaned. Pillow casings, bed sheets, and clothing should be washed in hot water (over 130°F). You can vacuum furniture, rugs, and carpeting if these recently touched your child's head. Keep in mind that lice can't live longer than about 48 hours when they are off someone's head. Pets and animals do not have to be checked; human head lice only like humans.

*

> Head lice are not dangerous, and they do not transmit diseases. Over-the-counter and prescription products can usually kill head lice, and they are mostly safe. It is important to use each product exactly as the package label states. The different products are used differently.

DIARRHEA

My 3-year-old son is having a lot of watery diarrhea. Are there any medicines I can buy to stop his diarrhea?

The answer is no. Although some antidiarrheal medicines (for example, Imodium) are advertised as being able to stop diarrhea, they should not be given to children. Imodium (loperamide) is available as a children's product, but I don't believe that it should be given to children. Another popular medicine for diarrhea or upset stomachs is Pepto-Bismol. Pepto-Bismol contains bismuth subsalicylate. Because bismuth subsalicylate is chemically similar to aspirin, Pepto-Bismol is best not given to children when they have viral infections, such as influenza or chicken pox. A product called Children's Pepto is also available and does not contain bismuth subsalicylate. It contains calcium carbonate, which is an antacid and will not treat diarrhea. Sometimes antidiarrheal medicines can be given to adults, but as I have stated throughout this book, *children are not small adults*. There are differences in how we use medicines in children as compared to adults. These antidiarrheal medicines can cause a blockage in a child's intestinal tract, which may be dangerous, even deadly.

The type of diarrhea I discuss here, and the type that is most common in children, is called *acute gastroenteritis*. In acute gastroenteritis, diarrhea comes on suddenly, it eventually goes away naturally, and it is not due to another serious medical problem. Many types of germs may cause diarrhea in children, but viruses are usually the cause. These "stomach bugs," as we often call them, change the way stool is formed in the intestinal tract and cause the sufferer to lose a lot of fluid (water). Some types of bacteria and parasites may also cause diarrhea in children, but not as often as viruses. Because viruses mostly cause diarrhea in children, antibiotics are not necessary or helpful. Sometimes diarrhea in children may be more serious, which means that the child needs to see a doctor right away or may need to go to a hospital. These situations include a child who has blood in the diarrhea or a very high fever (100.4°F or above for infants younger than 3 months, or 102.2°F or above for infants 3 months or older) or a child who has other serious medical conditions.

It is important that parents understand that the main danger with diarrhea in an infant or child is the loss of fluid (water) and electrolytes. Electrolytes are sodium, potassium, and chloride. The more watery a child's diarrhea is, the more fluid and electrolytes he or she is losing. A child who loses too much water and electrolytes may become dangerously ill and even die. Diarrhea and dehydration is a major killer of young children (younger than 5 years old) in the world, mostly in underdeveloped countries with poor medical care. Each year about 2 million young children worldwide die from diarrhea and dehydration. In the United States, about 300 children die each year from diarrhea and dehydration. So when your child has diarrhea, try not to focus on stopping the diarrhea, although we certainly want the diarrhea to stop. Focus instead on preventing your child from becoming dehydrated. Usually the diarrhea will eventually stop naturally.

How can I tell if my son is dehydrated?

When your child has diarrhea you need to be in contact with your child's doctor. You may not have to bring your son into the doctor's office, and the doctor's office may not want a child ill with infectious diarrhea in their waiting room, where the infection could easily spread to other children. If your son is not too sick, you can take

TABLE 6.1   Changes in a child's body with dehydration

BODY CHANGE	MILD-MODERATE DEHYDRATION	SEVERE DEHYDRATION
Alertness or behavior	Irritable; restless; tired	Unconscious; very tired or lethargic
Thirst	Thirsty; wants to drink	Drinks poorly; unable to drink
Breathing	Normal or fast	Deep breathing
Tears	Decreased	None
Mouth	Dry	Very dry or parched
Urine	Decreased urine	Decreased or hardly any urine

care of him at home, calling your doctor's office on the phone for help and directions.

As I described above, when a child has diarrhea, you must take steps to prevent dehydration and to rehydrate a child who is dehydrated. How do you tell if your child is dehydrated? Doctors describe dehydration in a child as "mild, moderate, or severe." Table 6.1 lists how a child's body changes with the severity of dehydration. When you call your child's doctor's office, they will ask you questions about how your child is feeling, such as how alert he is or how often he is urinating. This helps the doctor determine if your child is dehydrated and, if so, the level of dehydration.

If my son is dehydrated, do I need to bring him to the hospital?

Many parents, and even some doctors, might want a child with "moderate" dehydration to go to a hospital or hospital emergency room for intravenous fluids. However, this isn't always necessary. Many medical studies have shown, and professional medical organizations such as the American Academy of Pediatrics and the Centers for Disease Control and Prevention have stated, that most children with mild and moderate dehydration can be treated at home with oral fluids, called oral rehydration solutions (ORS). Using ORS can work just as well as intravenous (IV) fluids to reduce dehydration in many children. Why bring your child to a hospital where he will most likely have an IV line placed, which means using a painful needle, when you can treat him in your own home?

Where can I buy oral rehydration solution for my son?
Can I use his favorite drink, apple juice, instead?

You can buy oral rehydration solutions in a pharmacy and other stores, such as many grocery stores or larger convenience stores (such as Target or K-Mart). A common brand name is Pedialyte (see table 6.2). These products also come as generic forms, which are usually cheaper. They come in either unflavored or flavored solutions, such as bubble gum, grape, and others. They are even available as freezer pops for older children. I have tasted some of these products, including the unflavored and flavored solutions. I thought the unflavored solution tasted terrible, and I don't recommend using it. The flavored solutions tasted better and improve when they are cold (so store them in your refrigerator).

Even though your son likes apple juice and apple juice is fluid, you should not give this to him, because apple juice can make your son's diarrhea worse, and he can lose more fluid. This is because juices contain a lot of sugar, and a large amount of sugar can pull more water from his body into the diarrheal fluid. Also, apple juice doesn't have enough sodium, potassium, or chloride to replace the electrolytes he lost in the diarrhea. A too low level of these electrolytes in the body can be dangerous.

It's best not to use sports drinks, such as Gatorade, either, as these sports drinks have too much sugar for a dehydrated child. And don't give your child plain water. Because plain water doesn't have electrolytes in it, giving plain water could cause the levels of these electrolytes in your child's body to become even more dangerously low. The oral rehydration solutions contain just the right amount of glucose (sugar) and electrolytes that his body needs to replace what was lost in diarrhea. Oral rehydration solutions are the only fluids that you should give your child if he is dehydrated or has diarrhea. It's a good idea always to keep some in your home, as you never know when diarrhea will strike. Your son's next episode of diarrhea may happen on a Sunday night at 1:00 a.m., when most pharmacies are closed.

I spoke to my child's doctor, and he said I could give my son Pedialyte at home. I went to the store and bought some—should I put it in his favorite cup and let him drink as much as he can?

No. If your son is thirsty, it may seem like a good idea to let him drink as much as he wants. However, if he drinks a lot of oral rehydration solution at one time, he'll probably throw it right back up. This happened to my son when he was younger and was ill and dehydrated. I filled up his sippy cup with fruit-flavored Pedialyte (red colored) and let him drink from it. He drank the full cup, and a few minutes

TABLE 6.2   Oral rehydration products

PRODUCT	COMES AS	COMMENTS
Pedialyte	• Liquid—flavored and unflavored • Freezer pops for older children • Powder packs	• Flavored tastes much better than unflavored. • Various flavors—grape, bubble gum, strawberry, fruit. • Keep in refrigerator and use cold (tastes better).
CeraLyte	• Powder packs • Liquid	• Different strengths (amount of sodium) and different flavors. • Not in most pharmacies, but available online.
Generic brands	• Liquid—flavored and unflavored	• Less expensive than brand name products. • Flavored probably tastes better than unflavored.

later, he threw it up all over a white T-shirt I had on (which was then stained bright red). The best way to give oral rehydration solution is to offer a little bit (1 to 2 teaspoonsful, or about 1/2 ounce) and to give this amount frequently (about every 5 to 10 minutes). So, as tempting as it might be, don't fill up your son's sippy cup or another cup and let him drink as much as he can, even if he is thirsty.

Your child's doctor will probably tell you how much oral rehydration solution to give your son, depending on how dehydrated he is and how much he weighs. If your son has mild dehydration, he would need about 25 ounces of oral rehydration solution to rehydrate him. This should be given over 3 to 4 hours, and not all at one time. Once he is rehydrated with these 25 ounces, he would need about 5 ounces of oral rehydration solution each time he has diarrhea, to prevent him from becoming dehydrated again.

My neighbor once told me that I could make my own rehydration solution to give my son. Can I use this if I run out of the oral rehydration solution I bought at the store?

There are recipes on how to make homemade rehydration solutions for children with diarrhea. I believe it is best to use commercially prepared solutions, but if you run out of hydration solution you bought at a store, or if you can't get to a store, you can make hydration solution at home. When making these solutions, be very careful and follow the directions exactly, as it is very easy to make a mistake when preparing them. If you make the solution incorrectly, you could potentially worsen your child's diarrhea and dehydration. For these recipes, go to www.rehydrate.org.

My son drank the rehydration solution, and he seems to be perking up. He hasn't eaten in awhile. Can he eat now?

Yes. Some parents may believe that a child shouldn't eat until diarrhea has completely stopped, but this is not true. If an infant with diarrhea is breast-fed, then the infant should continue to nurse as normal. Infants who are formula-fed should be given formula as normal after they have been rehydrated. Do not dilute the formula; the same formula should be given as when the infant doesn't have diarrhea. Most infants do not need a lactose-free formula (lactose is a type of sugar in milk and milk-based products). Older children, such as your 3-year-old, can continue to eat their normal diet, and they should eat as normal. Some people say to wait at least 24 hours after diarrhea starts to feed a child, but this is not true, and waiting can actually make diarrhea last longer. It's best to avoid some foods, however, as these foods may make your son's diarrhea worse: soft drinks, juices, gelatin desserts, and other foods with a lot of sugar in them. You may hear about special diets for children with diarrhea, such as the BRAT diet. BRAT stands for bananas, rice, applesauce, and toast. While these foods are easier for your child to digest, they may not provide enough calories. Foods you can give your child include potatoes, wheat, bread, cereal, rice, lean meat, yogurt, and vegetables. So, allow your child to eat what he normally does, with the exception of drinks and foods that have a lot of sugar in them, which should be avoided.

> Viruses cause most cases of diarrhea in children, and antibiotics are not necessary. Dehydration and electrolyte loss is what can make diarrhea potentially dangerous. Use special oral rehydration solutions to rehydrate your child. Children with diarrhea should continue to have their normal diet, except high-sugar drinks and foods.

CONSTIPATION

My 2-year-old daughter hasn't pooped in two days.
What is the best medicine to give for her constipation?

Parents and doctors often have different definitions of constipation in children. Many parents believe that their child should have a bowel movement every day, but this is not necessarily true. Bowel habits differ among children, and what is normal for one child may be abnormal for another. A medical definition of constipation in children is a stool frequency of fewer than three bowel movements per week. Constipation can also be defined as a delay or difficulty in pooping for two weeks or more, or bowel movements that are painful or when stool is retained (kept inside the bowel, and not completely evacuated). As your daughter hasn't pooped in two days, this may not mean that she is constipated. It depends on what she has eaten recently and what her activity level has been.

It's now been four days since my daughter last pooped. Today she finally pooped a lot, but it was painful, and she was crying. I called our pediatrician, and he told us to get Milk of Magnesia to give her every day. Is this a good medicine for a 2-year-old?

There are several laxative medicines that can be used safely in children. These medicines have been used and studied a lot in children, and we know that they work well. Most of them you can buy in a pharmacy without a prescription (over the counter). These medicines include mineral oil, magnesium hydroxide (Milk of Magnesia is a common brand name), lactulose, and sorbitol. Some children who are constipated may need to be disimpacted first. This means that the child has a large amount of stool that is impacting the rectum (think of this like a sink drain that is plugged up). Once the impaction is cleared, the child often will need to be given a laxative every day as maintenance treatment of constipation.

Magnesium hydroxide is a good medicine for a 2-year-old, and it should work well to prevent constipation in your daughter. The amount of magnesium hydroxide your pediatrician wants your daughter to have may be more than what is listed on the bottle directions.

More of this medicine is often necessary when treating constipation in children. Another medicine that many doctors like to use when treating constipation in children is polyethylene glycol, commonly known as MiraLax. This medicine is also available generically. The label of a bottle of polyethylene glycol states that MiraLax should only be used in adults. Polyethylene glycol has been studied in many children, however, and it is safe and it works very well. As I discuss in chapter 1, the directions and package label for some medicines state "for use in adults only" because the company that makes the medicine has not formally tested it in children. This doesn't necessarily mean that the medicine is dangerous for children. (This should not be interpreted to mean that any medication labeled "for use in adults only" can be given to children. You should give such medications to children only on the advice of your child's doctor.) Other researchers may have tested the medicine in children and found it to be safe and to work well. This is what has occurred for polyethylene glycol. I believe that it is safe to use in children, and I've spoken with many parents who have told me that it works well and that it is easy to give to children.

Some parents may believe that giving polyethylene glycol to their child for many months may cause him or her to become "addicted" to this medicine. This is not true. Some children with constipation may need medicine for many months or even years. The medicines I discuss above are not "addicting," but some children continue to need the medicines to have regular and normal bowel movements. When the medicines are no longer needed, they may be stopped without difficulty. Talk to your child's doctor before you use polyethylene glycol or any of the laxatives I discuss here to be sure that your child uses the best medicine for her.

If magnesium hydroxide works well to prevent constipation in your daughter, there is a good chance that she may need to take this medicine for at least several years. Several long-term studies of children with constipation have shown that many children needed to take a laxative for several years or longer before they could stop the medicine and not be constipated.

Some laxatives should not be given to young infants (younger than 12 months), and they shouldn't be used a lot for children. Don't give mineral oil to young infants, as they can choke when swallowing it; if this happens, the mineral oil may damage an infant's lungs. If a young infant is constipated, glycerin suppositories or barley malt extract are often used as laxatives. Some laxatives are called stimulant laxatives, such as bisacodyl (a brand name is Dulcolax) or senna. These medicines can be given to children, but they are best used only occasionally and they shouldn't be used every day for many days together.

---

*

Constipation is common in children. Several medicines have been shown to be safe and work well in infants and children. You can buy some of these medicines without a doctor's prescription. Many children need to take a laxative for several years or more for constipation.

PAIN MEDICINES

In this short section I discuss two common medicines that can be used for treating pain and discomfort in children. Young children may have pain from everything from ear infections (for more about medicine for pain from ear infections, see chapter 4) to a skinned knee. The type of pain children are probably most afraid of, however, is pain from a shot at the doctor's office. I discuss how you can reduce this type of pain and comfort your child during shots in chapter 1.

My 8-year-old son was riding his bike this morning, and he fell and hurt his knee. Fortunately, he was wearing his helmet. He says his knee hurts, and now it looks swollen. I have Tylenol and Motrin at home. Is one better than the other for his pain?

You can use either acetaminophen (such as Tylenol) or ibuprofen (such as Motrin or Advil). Both of these medicines work well for pain in children. Ibuprofen may be better for your son now, however, because ibuprofen is an anti-inflammatory medicine, which means that it treats swelling. Acetaminophen treats pain, but it doesn't treat swelling. If your son's knee wasn't swollen, you could give him either acetaminophen or ibuprofen.

When giving acetaminophen or ibuprofen to children, whether for pain or fever, it may be very easy to make a mistake and give too much or not enough medicine. As I discuss in chapter 3, acetaminophen is a safe medicine when it is given correctly. But if too much acetaminophen is accidentally given to a child, it may be very dangerous and even deadly. Too much ibuprofen is not as dangerous as too much acetaminophen, but you certainly don't want to give too much ibuprofen, either. (Chapter 3 explains how to measure these medications correctly.) But it is easy to make a mistake and accidentally give too much (or too little) of these medicines. Here's why:

- *Different types and strengths.* Acetaminophen and ibuprofen both come in different types and strengths (how much medicine is in each tablet or liquid). They come as products for children and for adults; for children, they also come in different strengths, so it can be easy to use the wrong strength accidentally.

- *Other medicines.* Many other medicines, especially over-the-counter medicines, have acetaminophen as one of their active ingredients. If you are not aware of this, you may accidentally give too much acetaminophen if you are using several different products at the same time.

- *Prescription pain medicines.* Some pain medicines prescribed by a doctor to treat a child's pain, such as liquid codeine products, also contain acetaminophen. If you are also giving plain Tylenol, you may accidentally give too much acetaminophen.

- *Measuring liquid medicine.* It is easy to make a mistake when measuring out liquid acetaminophen or ibuprofen, and you may accidentally give too much or too little medicine (see chapter 3).

- *More is not better.* Acetaminophen or ibuprofen may not make a child's pain go away completely, so it may be tempting to give more medicine. Nevertheless, do not give acetaminophen more than five times in 24 hours or ibuprofen more than four times in 24 hours.

✳

Acetaminophen and ibuprofen both work well for treating pain in children. Ibuprofen also treats inflammation or swelling, while acetaminophen does not. Both acetaminophen and ibuprofen are safe medicines when they are used correctly, but it can be easy to give too much acetaminophen or ibuprofen accidentally. Too much acetaminophen is dangerous for children.

ASTHMA: HELPING YOUR CHILD BREATHE NORMALLY

Asthma is the most common chronic medical condition in children. About 7 million children—close to 10 percent of all children—in the United States have asthma. There are several types of asthma, and for all types, many different medicines can help children breathe better. Asthma may be very dangerous. It even can cause death. Many prescription medicines are available for children with asthma, and if these medicines are used correctly, a child with asthma should be able to do everything that other children do. The section that follows warns about the many ways these medicines may be used incorrectly and offers advice on how to use asthma medicines the right way.

My 10-year-old son has asthma, and he uses several medicines, two of which he takes every day. Our doctor told us today that my 5-year-old daughter also has asthma, but she only needs to use an inhaler when she doesn't feel good. Why do they take different medicines if they both have asthma?

Probably your children are using different medicines because they have different types of asthma. There are two main types of asthma: *intermittent* and *persistent*. Intermittent asthma means that a child may have breathing problems only at certain times or seasons, such as during the spring and fall, when allergies more commonly occur, or only when she has a cold. During other times or seasons, such as summer or winter, a child with intermittent asthma may not have any breathing problems related to asthma at all. A child with intermittent asthma usually uses medicine only when she needs it to help overcome breathing difficulties; she doesn't usually need to use medicine daily.

A child with persistent asthma has breathing problems nearly all year. If this child does not use daily medicines, he may have breathing problems nearly any time and daily, or most days of a week. A child with intermittent asthma has breathing difficulties fewer than two days per week on average, while a child with persistent asthma has breathing difficulties two or more days per week on average. It sounds like your daughter has intermittent asthma and your son has persistent asthma.

It's been about five weeks since my 10-year-old son started using his Flovent inhaler. He is feeling much better and his breathing has been good. Our doctor didn't tell us how long he should use Flovent. Since he is feeling better now, can he stop using his Flovent?

You should continue to give your son Flovent unless your doctor tells you to stop it. Some medicines for asthma should be given daily, even when the child feels better and is not having any breathing problems. Medicines such as Flovent are called long-term controllers, which means they help to control asthma over weeks, months, and years. These preventative-type medicines keep asthma from worsening and help a child breathe normally.

Stopping preventive medicines when a child with asthma feels better is a common mistake parents make. I've seen this happen many times. It's tempting and easy to do—after all, why continue to give your child a medicine when he is doing well? The reason is that asthma is a chronic disease, and the type of asthma your son has— persistent asthma—means that the problem in his lungs (inflammation and swelling) is always there and needs to be controlled every day. Flovent is an excellent medicine to do this, but it must be given every day, even when your son feels good.

There are two types of medicines used to treat asthma: *quick-relief* and *long-term controllers*. Quick-relief medicines treat breathing problems that are happening right now. The generic name of the most commonly used quick-relief medicine is albuterol; some trade names of albuterol are ProAir, Ventolin, and Proventil. Another commonly used quick-relief medicine is levalbuterol (Xopenex). Albuterol and levalbuterol work very quickly, within several minutes, to relax, or open up, the airways in the lungs to let more air in to help the child breathe better. I tell parents that these medicines "un-crimp" the garden hose (airways in the lungs) to allow more "water" (air and oxygen) to flow out. Quick-relief medicines should be used only when a child has trouble breathing. If the child is doing well, they don't have to be used. We say that they are used "as needed." Sometimes, albuterol and levalbuterol can be used preventatively, such as just before exercise to prevent breathing problems during physical activity. Mostly, however, they are used as needed, and if a child is not having breathing problems, they don't have to be used.

The other type of medicine, long-term controllers, may be thought of as the "opposite" of quick-relief medicines. Long-term controllers don't work quickly for breathing problems happening right now, and they should be taken every day to help control asthma long term, even if the child is doing well. These medicines include inhaled corticosteroids such as Flovent, Advair, or QVAR, and another popular medicine, Singulair. They should be used ev-

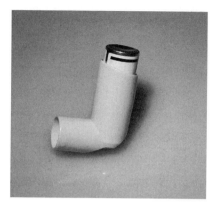

One type of inhaler
for treating asthma.

ery day, even when the child's asthma is well controlled. If the child is doing well, then these long-term control medicines are probably working well.

✱

There are two types of medicines for asthma: quick-relief medicines and long-term controller medicines. Quick-relief medicines work within a few minutes to help immediate breathing difficulties, and they should be used only when needed. Long-term controller medicines work slowly, and they help to prevent breathing difficulties. They should be taken every day, even when your child is breathing normally. Be sure you know which type of medicines your child has and when to use them.

When my son started using his Flovent inhaler, we were told that this was a steroid medicine. I am worried about him using a steroid medicine for a long time. Don't steroid medicines have a lot of side effects?

Yes, steroid medicines (also called corticosteroids) may have a lot of side effects, and some of these side effects may be dangerous. However—and this is important—these side effects depend on how the medicine is given (whether as a tablet or liquid or inhaled by a nebulizer or inhaler) and the dose (how much medicine is given). The most important factor for your son is that his Flovent is inhaled and not a tablet or liquid. When inhaler medicines such as Flovent are used, although some of the medicine goes to other areas of the body, most of it stays in the lungs. When someone takes a steroid such as prednisone as a tablet or liquid, then the medicine is absorbed into the bloodstream and travels all over the body, which is how the many side effects of steroids occur. Because Flovent stays mostly in the lungs, this form of steroid doesn't have the long list of side effects that prednisone and other oral steroids do.

As discussed in chapter 1, all medicines have side effects. Flovent is no exception. The most common side effects of Flovent (and other inhaled steroid medicines) are a change in voice sound (what the child sounds like when he or she talks) and thrush (a fungal infection in the mouth). Neither of these side effects is dangerous, and both may easily be prevented or treated. A side effect that may be more serious from an inhaled steroid medicine, but is much less likely to occur, is a potential to decrease a child's growth velocity (how much they grow in height and how fast). Several medical studies have shown that inhaled steroids may decrease a child's height velocity and that these effects mostly occur in the first year of using the medicine; after that, the child is likely to grow normally. And, it is very likely that a child's final height as an adult will be normal. In these studies, when the child's height was affected, the average decrease in growth rate was minimal—about half an inch. Asthma that is not treated or is not well controlled can also decrease a child's growth and height.

There are several things you can do to reduce or eliminate these side effects. One is to use a spacer device with the Flovent inhaler (see below for more about spacer devices). Another is to get your son to rinse his mouth out and spit after he uses his Flovent; mouth rinsing helps prevent any of the medicine in the mouth from being swallowed, where it can then travel to other parts of the body to cause more side effects. I tell parents to brush the child's teeth and then have the child rinse and spit after using inhaled steroids such as Flovent. Your child's height will be measured at each doctor's appointment. If your child's growth is less than normal because of

the Flovent (which is unlikely), then the doctor may prescribe another medicine instead. Your child's doctor will also try to reduce
the Flovent dose to the lowest amount of medicine needed to control
your child's asthma. This also reduces the likelihood that his growth
will be affected by the medication.

The side effects of inhaled steroids, such as Flovent, are a good
example of the *benefit* of a medicine versus its *risk*, as I discussed in
chapter 1. Inhaled steroid medicines are the best type of medicine we
have for controlling asthma. There are other types of medicines to
control asthma, but they often don't work as well. The risks of using
inhaled steroid medicines are the side effects discussed above. For
most children, I believe that the benefits of inhaled steroids—to control asthma (a potentially very dangerous medical condition)—are
greater than these risks. For a small number of children (for example
if a child's height is affected), a parent may believe that the risks out-
weigh the benefits. This is a reasonable conclusion, and a doctor can
prescribe other medicines to try to control the child's asthma.

*My son has been using his Flovent twice a day, every day. He hadn't
had any breathing problems, until a few days ago. For the past few days
he has been coughing a lot, and he is having some trouble breathing.
We went to our pediatrician, and he prescribed prednisone tablets for
10 days. My son also had prednisone about 6 weeks ago for breathing
problems. Is all of this prednisone safe? Doesn't prednisone have a lot
of dangerous side effects?*

Prednisone, a steroid medicine, may have many side effects. However, the most dangerous side effects only happen when prednisone
is taken for a longer time. In this case a "longer time" usually means
two weeks or more. The list of these potential dangerous side effects
is long and includes increasing risk of infection, stunting of growth,
weakened bones and bone fractures, and cataracts in the eyes. If your
son takes prednisone for one 10-day period, these side effects will
not happen. These effects may occur if a child takes a lot of prednisone over the course of a year, even if it is given at separate times.

A child would probably have to have about 30–40 days of prednisone altogether over the course of one year for these side effects to occur. So, if your son had prednisone 6 weeks ago (for 10 days) and then has another 10 days of prednisone, this would not be enough time for these side effects to occur.

Prednisone may also have "short-term" side effects, meaning that some side effects may occur on the first day or so of taking prednisone. While these side effects are not dangerous, they may be frustrating to parents. I've spoken with many parents whose children have had these side effects from prednisone, and they can be quite bothersome. Perhaps most concerning to parents is the effect of prednisone on a child's behavior. Prednisone may cause children to be moody or grumpy, to cry more easily, and even to be more aggressive. One mother told me that her child was biting other children when taking prednisone. Prednisone may cause children to have more energy, be hyperactive, and not sleep well. It may also increase a child's appetite. Not all children taking prednisone will have these side effects, and some may not have any of these side effects. What can be done if these side effects occur? If these side effects do happen when your child is taking prednisone, don't stop giving it unless you speak with your child's doctor first. A doctor can lower the dose of prednisone, which may help decrease these side effects. Once prednisone is stopped, the side effects should go away quickly.

Is my son's prednisone the same type of steroid I read about in the newspaper that some athletes take to perform better in sports?

No. The steroids that some athletes take—which are illegal to use in sports—are different types of steroids from prednisone, which is a corticosteroid. The steroids that get athletes in trouble are called anabolic steroids. *Anabolic* means that they build up muscles and have other effects. Anabolic steroids are very similar chemically to testosterone, the male sex hormone. Anabolic steroids have many side effects, and they are not the same as prednisone and other steroid medicines used to treat asthma.

*

Steroid medicines when given by mouth as a liquid or tablet may cause a lot of side effects, and some of these side effects can be dangerous. However, the dangerous side effects don't happen when using steroids for a few days. When steroids are inhaled into the lungs, most of these dangerous side effects don't happen. Steroid medicines inhaled in the lungs are the most effective type of medicine to control asthma. If your child uses steroid medicines, ask your doctor and pharmacist about these side effects and what you can do to reduce the chances they will occur.

I took my 5-year-old daughter to our pediatrician for a check-up visit about her asthma. She is doing well, and the doctor told me that she could use an inhaler for her albuterol instead of using the nebulizer. Isn't she too young to use an inhaler? Does an inhaler work as well as a nebulizer?

Asthma is a medical condition of the lungs, so it is best if the medicines we use to treat asthma are given into the lungs. There are several ways to give medicines to the lungs. Most parents are probably familiar with using a nebulizer to deliver medicine to the lungs. There are different types of nebulizers, and they all turn a liquid medicine into an aerosol (an aerosol is very small drops of liquid in a gas). By turning liquid medicine into an aerosol, nebulizers are able to deliver medicine more easily into the lungs, where it treats asthma. Nebulizers may be used for all ages—newborn infants, older children, and adults. Nebulizers can be very useful, but they have some disadvantages. They are bulky to carry, they need a source of power (electricity or a battery), and it may take 10 minutes or more to deliver all of the medicine.

An inhaler is another way to give asthma medicine to infants and young children, and it is often much easier and quicker. Many asthma medicines come as inhalers, also known as puffers. There are different types of inhalers. The type of inhaler most commonly used is called a metered-dose inhaler (such as ProAir). This type of inhaler

TABLE 6.3 How to use a metered-dose inhaler (MDI) and spacer*

STEP	COMMENTS
Shake the inhaler a few times.	Of course, take the cap off.
Breathe out all the way.	I tell children to pretend that they are blowing out candles on a birthday cake.
Put the spacer in your mouth, with lips tight around it.**	• The inhaler should be in the other end of the spacer. • For infants or younger children, put a face mask on the spacer and place the mask over the face, with a tight seal on the face.
Press down on the inhaler and at the same time *slowly* and *deeply* breathe in.	• Breathe in slowly—over 3 to 5 seconds. • If using a face mask, the infant or child should breathe in and out normally into the face mask 5 or 6 times.
Take the spacer out of your mouth.	• Keep your lips closed and tight.
Hold your breath for 10 seconds, and then breathe out.	• Count to 10 in your head. • This is not necessary with a face mask.
If another puff is needed . . .	• For albuterol or levalbuterol, wait 30 seconds between puffs.

* There are several types of inhalers and spacers, and every inhaler may not work well with every spacer. These directions are for metered-dose inhalers, such as ProAir. Also see the directions that come with each type of inhaler and spacer.

** Some doctors may tell you that your child, especially if he or she is older, can use an inhaler without a spacer by spraying the inhaler into the mouth from 1 to 2 inches outside of the mouth or by placing the inhaler in the mouth. I believe that using an inhaler together with a spacer is better.

has a propellant in it, so when you press down on it, the medicine comes shooting out as a spray. Inhalers may also be given to infants and young children. How? We attach the inhaler to a spacer device, also called a holding chamber (some trade names are AeroChamber and Vortex). This spacer device briefly "holds" the medicine and allows the infant or child to breathe in the medicine when normally breathing. For infants and younger children, we also use a mask that attaches to the spacer. Different sizes of masks are available. The

✳

> Medicines for asthma can be given into the lungs using a nebulizer or inhaler for children and infants. These devices are used differently, and it is easy to use them incorrectly. Be sure you know the correct way to use the nebulizer or inhaler that your child has. Ask your pharmacist or doctor whether you are using a device correctly.

mask should form a tight seal on the infant's or child's face. He'll look like a jet pilot ready to take off!

I've found that many parents believe that a nebulizer works better than an inhaler for their child, and this may be true for that child. However, several medical studies have shown that inhalers work just as well as nebulizers at delivering medicine into the lungs to decrease breathing difficulties for asthma. Some hospital emergency departments use inhalers, and not nebulizers, to give medicine to an asthmatic child who is having breathing problems. I recommend inhalers frequently to parents because they are easy to use, they are much easier to carry than a nebulizer (an inhaler fits into a mother's purse or bag), and they don't need a source of power. Some doctors may tell you that a spacer is not necessary. But even if an older child uses an inhaler alone, a spacer device can still increase the amount of medicine that is delivered into the lungs (up to two or three times as much medicine).

Nebulizers, inhalers, and spacers must be used correctly. I've seen many children and parents who do not use nebulizers and inhalers the right way. If the devices are not used correctly, then only some of the medicine, and perhaps none of it, is delivered to the lungs, and the medicine will not be able to help your child's breathing. See table 6.3 for the correct way to use inhalers and spacers. A common mistake with using a nebulizer is to hold the tubing up against the child's nose and mouth and let him or her breathe in the aerosol medicine from the air. This doesn't work. Instead, if you have an infant or young child, then you should attach a face mask to the tube, similar to what is described above for using a spacer. When a child is old enough to take a slow, deep breath, then a face mask is no longer

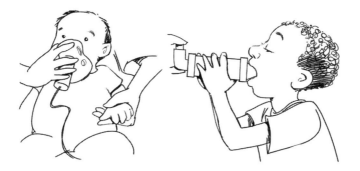

Either a nebulizer or an inhaler may be used to deliver medicine to an infant or child with asthma. It is important that these devices be used properly.

needed. Then the child can place the mouthpiece or nebulizer tubing in his or her mouth and inhale using slow, deep breaths. A common mistake I've seen children make with inhalers and spacers is breathing in too fast. Breathing too fast causes more of the medicine to stay in the mouth and not go to the lungs. If you are not sure whether your child is using the inhaler correctly, show your pharmacist or doctor how you are using it, and he or she will help you adjust so that you are doing it correctly.

ATTENTION-DEFICIT HYPERACTIVITY DISORDER (ADHD)

Attention-deficit hyperactivity disorder, or ADHD, is a common medical condition among children. Some people call ADHD by an older name, ADD (attention-deficit disorder). Between 3 and 9 million children have ADHD in the United States, about 4 to 12 percent of all children. Children with ADHD have difficulty controlling their behavior, mainly in three ways: *inattention* (they have trouble paying attention and are easily distracted), *hyperactivity* (they are constantly moving or talking), and *impulsivity* (they have trouble waiting, and they interrupt things and others). Nearly all children can have these behaviors sometimes. But when a child has ADHD, these behaviors are very noticeable and frequently cause problems in school or in how the child behaves with other children. Not every child with ADHD will have all of these behaviors, and there are different types of ADHD. We are not sure what causes ADHD, and there is no cure for it. However, ADHD often can be well controlled with medicines and other treatments.

Our pediatrician told me today that my 6-year-old son has ADHD. He can't seem to sit still, and he is constantly on the go. Our pediatrician told me he wants my son to start taking a stimulant medicine. That doesn't make sense! How can a stimulant medicine help a child who is hyperactive? Are all medicines for ADHD stimulants?

It does seem strange that a stimulant medicine is used to treat ADHD, when many children with ADHD are hyperactive. Just as we don't know exactly what causes ADHD, we also don't know exactly how the stimulant medicines work to control it. There are two main types of stimulant medicines: methylphenidate (some trade names are Ritalin, Concerta, Focalin, and Daytrana) and amphetamine (some trade names are Dexedrine, Adderall, and Vyvanse). We do know that the stimulant medicines work well for most children with ADHD. About 80 percent of children with ADHD will improve with a stimulant medicine, and many medical studies have shown that stimulants help to control ADHD. Most of the medicines we use to treat ADHD are stimulants. One medicine also commonly used, however, is not a stimulant medicine—atomoxetine (Strattera). Although Strattera can also work well to treat ADHD, for many children it does not work as well as the stimulant medicines.

We started our 6-year-old son on Ritalin, which is a stimulant medicine. It seems to be helping. When I called the pharmacy for a refill, they told us that this medicine doesn't have refills and that we need to call or visit our pediatrician again. Why?

Ritalin and all of the stimulant medicines are controlled substances, which means that the amount of medicine a doctor can prescribe and a pharmacist can dispense is "controlled" to only a specified amount. You can only have refills by getting another prescription. The reason for this is not because the stimulant medicines are dangerous for your son to take. It is because Ritalin and other stimulant medicines have a high potential for abuse by those not taking it for medical purposes. People who don't have ADHD, such as college students or adults who work long hours or work at night, may take stimulant medicines illegally (without a prescription from a doctor) to help them stay focused or awake. Because the stimulant medicines have the potential to be abused this way, it's best to control how much medicine is dispensed from the pharmacy. Ritalin is a controlled medicine to help make sure it is used for the person and purpose it was prescribed; "controlled" does not mean that the medicine is dangerous for your son.

Our pediatrician didn't tell us how long our son would be taking Ritalin. Will he have to take it for a long time? I've read that Ritalin is addicting. Is this true?

How long children with ADHD need to continue taking stimulant medicine will vary. If a child taking Ritalin has improved, it is likely that the child will continue to take Ritalin for a while. Many children with ADHD continue to have ADHD as adolescents and even adults. As long as a stimulant medicine is helping a child with ADHD, it usually is continued. As children get older, some of their hyperactivity and impulsivity may decrease. Sometimes doctors will try to stop a stimulant medicine after several years, especially during the summer when the child is not in school, to see if medicine is still necessary. If the child's ADHD becomes difficult to control without the medicine, this is proof that the medicine should be continued.

Ritalin and other stimulant medicines are not addicting. As I explain above, the reason why the amount of medicine you can get at the pharmacy with a prescription is limited is the potential for abuse by others, not by the person using it to treat ADHD. There are many medical studies that show that adolescents with ADHD who take stimulant medicine are *less likely* to get into trouble using illegal drugs such as cocaine. This is because stimulants help to control ADHD and its associated behaviors, such as impulsive behavior. An adolescent whose ADHD is well controlled by taking a stimulant medicine is less likely to be impulsive and begin using illegal drugs.

I'm worried about the side effects of Ritalin, especially if my son has to take it for many years. A neighbor told me that Ritalin can stunt a child's growth. Is this true?

Ritalin and the stimulant medicines have the potential for side effects, as do all medicines. The more common side effects that Ritalin and stimulant medicines may cause include decreased appetite (sometimes weight loss also), headaches, stomach pain, and trouble sleeping. Most of the time these side effects are not bothersome, and the child may continue to take the medicine. Rarely, stimulant medicines may cause a child to have hallucinations. Sometimes these side effects will go away slowly. Giving the medicine with food will often avoid the decreased appetite and headache side effects. The many different stimulant products work for different lengths of time. Some stimulant products last only 3 to 4 hours, while others can last up to 12 hours. Your child's doctor may try to use a product that lasts longer, which may help to reduce some of these side effects.

Some medical studies show that stimulant medicines may slow a child's growth. If a stimulant medicine does affect a child's growth, it is likely to be a small amount. These studies have shown that a slowing of growth of about half an inch per year may occur within the first three years of taking the medicine. Several studies that have followed children as they got older found that their adult heights were not affected by medicine. Your child's doctor should measure your child's height each time he is seen in the office.

The side effects of the stimulant medicines are another good example of the point I discussed in chapter 1 about the benefits and risks of medicines. For most children with ADHD, there are many benefits of using stimulant medicines. Stimulant medicines can allow children to perform better in school. The medicines can potentially help them not only get better grades but also develop important social skills (such as how to get along with other children and teachers). This is important developmentally. The risks of using stimulant medicines are the side effects discussed above. For many children, the benefits are probably much greater than the risks of these medicines.

CHAPTER 7

Where Can I Find More Information about My Child's Medicines?

Information about children's medicines and medical conditions that affect children is widely available. One of the best sources of information is your pharmacist. Later in this chapter I discuss how you can get the best and most useful information from your pharmacist. You can also find medical information in your local bookstore, library, or online bookstore.

Perhaps the easiest place to look, of course, is on the Internet. There are thousands of Web sites containing information about medicines and medical conditions. Only some of these sites are reliable, however. Reliable information is medically accurate and up-to-date. The purpose of a reliable Web site is mostly to educate you, not to sell you something. Several recent studies have shown that many medical Web sites contain inaccurate medical information or information that is not up-to-date. Medical information changes very quickly, and a site that has not been updated recently may contain inaccurate information. In this chapter, I discuss how you can judge whether a Web site is likely to be reliable. I also list many Web sites that I believe are reliable and that you can use as a source of medical information.

This chapter will help you answer these questions:

- How can I tell whether a medical Web site is accurate and reliable?

- What are good medical Web sites I can use regularly?

- Where can I find other sources of information, including good books, about children's medicines?

- What questions should I ask my pharmacist about my child's medicines?

- What questions should I ask my child's doctor about my child's medicines?

I am looking on the Internet for information about my son's Ritalin. There are so many Web sites about Ritalin. How can I tell which are reliable?

The characteristics of a reliable Web site are listed in table 7.1. The characteristics of an unreliable Web site are listed in table 7.2. A reliable Web site provides medically accurate, up-to-date, and unbiased information about children's health and medicines. Its primary purpose is to educate or inform you, not to sell you a product.

It is easy to be misled into thinking that a Web site is reliable based on its appearance. A Web site that is colorful, flashy, and fun to look at isn't necessarily one that will provide reliable information about medicines and health conditions. Be sure to look beyond the flash and fun for evidence (as described in table 7.1) that the site offers accurate and up-to-date medical information.

If you type "Ritalin" into a common Internet search engine such as Yahoo or Google, you will get results for thousands of different sites. Looking at all, or even most, of these Web sites would be impossible, so you want to start with several trusted sites. For information on topics about children's medications or health conditions, you usually can start with the same few organizations' Web sites:

- the American Academy of Pediatrics (www.aap.org), the professional medical organization of pediatricians,

- the Centers for Disease Control and Prevention (www.cdc.gov), the U.S. government agency on national health issues, and

- the Food and Drug Administration (www.fda.gov), the U.S. government agency that regulates medicine use and safety.

TABLE 7.1 Characteristics of a reliable Web site

AREA	WHAT TO LOOK FOR
About us	• Look for a statement describing the purpose of the Web site. It should be to inform the public, not to sell something.
Reviewed by	• Information on the site should be written and reviewed by health professionals.
Last updated	• Look for a recent date. Because medical information changes so rapidly, the Web site should be updated frequently.
Contact us, Help, or Ask a question	• You should be able to contact someone at the Web site to ask a question.
Advertisements	• Advertisements should be clearly labeled as advertisements. • Information and writing on the site should not frequently suggest that you buy a product.
Privacy statement	• If personal information is requested, the site should display a policy about how this information will be used.
Site address (URL)	• Web sites ending with ".org," ".edu," or ".gov" are more likely to provide good medical information. • .org = organization (such as a professional medical organization).
References, Links, or Sources	• Medical facts and claims should be supported by published studies or by reference to another reliable Web site.
Sponsored by	• A Web site sponsored by an educational institution or professional medical organization is more likely to provide reliable information.
Search	• Searching within the Web site allows you to find more information. There should not be broken or dead-end links.

The primary purpose of a reliable Web site is to provide you with accurate, up-to-date, and unbiased medical information. It is not to sell you a product.

TABLE 7.2 Characteristics of an unreliable Web site

AREA	WHAT TO LOOK FOR
About us	• If the site was developed by just one or two people or by a commercial company, or if the information was written by someone whose identity cannot be clearly established, it may not be as reliable as other Web sites.
Reviewed by	• Information on a Web site that is not reviewed by health professionals is not as reliable.
Last updated	• If there is no indication of when the Web site was last reviewed, it is not as reliable.
Contact us, Help, or *Ask a question*	• If you can't contact anyone at the Web site, it is not as reliable.
Advertisements	• If advertisements are not labeled, and there are many advertisements on the site, it is not as reliable. If the information in the site frequently suggests that you buy a product, it is not as reliable.
Privacy statement	• If there is no privacy statement, or if it states that your information will be shared with other commercial companies, it is not as reliable.
Site address (URL)	• Web sites ending with ".com" are more likely trying to sell you something (although some hospitals have ".com" addresses and still provide good information). • .com = commercial.
References, Links, or *Sources*	• If medical information is given or claims are made about how good a medicine or product is without a reference to supporting evidence, or if information or claims sound too good to be true, it is not as reliable.
Sponsored by	• A Web site sponsored by a company is more likely biased toward certain commercial products and is not as reliable.
Product claims	• Web sites that promote "dramatic results," "breakthrough" treatments, or "cures" are not as reliable.

The primary purpose of an unreliable Web site is to sell you a product. A site is also considered unreliable if the information is biased to one opinion and is not medically accurate, up-to-date, or reliable. It is not meant to imply that the site does not have any purpose or use whatsoever.

These organizations' sites have information about medicines used for treating ADHD, including Ritalin, and they are written for the public, using nonmedical language. You can print off information, or you can order pamphlets or books (some at no cost) about ADHD and treatment. See table 7.3 for more Web sites about common medical conditions affecting children.

My infant son is almost 2 months old and is supposed to have his first set of immunizations in 3 weeks. I was curious what immunizations he will get, so I looked on the Internet. Some Web sites said vaccines are dangerous! What should I do?

As I discussed in chapter 5, some people believe that vaccines are dangerous and that children shouldn't receive them. I disagree with this, as do nearly all pediatricians. Probably the best (medically accurate and unbiased) Web site for information on children's vaccines is the Centers for Disease Control and Prevention: www.cdc.gov/vaccines. Use the *For Parents* link to reach the current immunization schedule for children. There you will find a readable description of the immunizations that are recommended for a 2-month-old infant. This site has links and information about immunization in children and specific vaccines (including safety and side effects) presented in nontechnical language for parents.

Instead of getting on the computer and looking on the Internet, are there any good books that I can use to quickly find more information about medicines?

I wrote this book because I could not find an up-to-date book that describes important issues on children's medications. There are, however, good books about specific medical topics and children, such as books on ADHD (attention-deficit hyperactivity disorder) or on vaccines (see chapter 5 for recommended books about children's vaccines). You can find books on medicines in general, such as *The Pill Book* and *The PDR Pocket Guide to Prescription Drugs* in your local bookstore. Although these books provide useful information about

TABLE 7.3 Web sites with information on children's medicines and medical conditions

WEB SITE	COMMENTS
www.aap.org	• The American Academy of Pediatrics is the professional medical organization of pediatricians. • Contains many useful links (*Parenting Corner, Health Topics*) about common medical conditions and medicines in nontechnical, easy-to-understand language. • Site visitors cannot email with specific questions about medicines (ask your pediatrician instead).
www.cdc.gov	• The Centers for Disease Control and Prevention is part of the U.S. government's Department of Health and Human Services. • Contains many useful links and information for numerous medical issues (children and adults).
www.cdc.gov/vaccines	• This area of the Centers for Disease Control and Prevention site is devoted to vaccines. • This is one of the best places for information on children's vaccines.
www.immunizationinfo.org	• Sponsored by the National Network for Immunization Information.
www.fda.gov/drugs	• The Food and Drug Administration is the U.S. government agency that regulates medicine use and safety. • See *Resources for You—Consumers*. • Useful for *Medication Guides*—information for specific medicines. • Useful for many issues about medicines.
www.kidsmeds.info	• The Pediatric Pharmacy Advocacy Group is a professional medical organization of pediatric pharmacists. • Contains much useful information on children's medicine issues, such as how to administer nose drops.
www.kidshealth.org	• Sponsored by the Nemours Foundation's Center for Children's Health. • Contains areas for *Parents, Kids*, and *Teens*. • Has a *Medications* area. • Site visitors can email with specific questions.
www.pharmacist.com	• The American Pharmacists Association is a professional organization of pharmacists. • See *Consumers* link. • Site is not specific to children.
www.medlineplus.org	• Sponsored by the National Library of Medicine. • See *About Your Health—Children*.
www.help4adhd.org	• Sponsored by the National Resource Center on ADHD. • Contains useful information about medicines and ADHD. • Visitors can email specific questions about ADHD.

many medicines, information about giving these medicines to children is covered only briefly, if at all. These books are probably most useful for adults who use many medicines. If you have a child with several medical conditions who requires many medicines, you may wish to look at these books to determine if they would be useful for you.

What questions about my child's medicine should I ask our pharmacist?

Your pharmacist can be one of the best sources of information about your child's medicines. Not only is your pharmacist knowledgeable about medicines, but he or she is also usually readily available to answer questions. Unlike with physicians, you don't need an appointment to ask your pharmacist a question. It may be difficult for the pharmacist to take time for questions when the pharmacy is busy. The busiest times in most community pharmacies are early mornings, late afternoons, Mondays and Fridays, and before holidays. A good time to call your pharmacist or ask your pharmacist a question in person is midweek and midafternoon. Many pharmacies are open 24 hours a day, so you can call these pharmacies any time.

Try to get to know one or two pharmacists at the pharmacy where you get prescriptions filled. If you develop a comfortable relationship with your pharmacists, you may feel more comfortable asking questions. If you don't like the pharmacists at your current pharmacy, find another pharmacy where you feel more comfortable. I believe that it is a good idea to use only one pharmacy for your child's medicines. This way the pharmacy will have a list of all the medicines your child takes, and the pharmacists can determine if any dangerous drug interactions may occur when any new medicines are added. If you use more than one pharmacy, the other pharmacy may not know all of the medicines your child is taking, and you may forget to tell them. Of course, your child's doctor should know about all of your child's medications and should avoid prescribing medicines that might interact in an unhealthy way.

I teach in a pharmacy school (Drake University College of Pharmacy in Des Moines, Iowa). Through the six years that our students spend with us, we teach them a great deal of information about many, many aspects of medicines and health care. When these students graduate, they know a lot about medicines. The same is true at other pharmacy schools. Take advantage of pharmacists' knowledge by asking them questions. When I work in the children's clinic, I want parents and children and adolescents to ask me questions about their medicines. I don't want them to leave the clinic with unanswered questions or unaddressed concerns about medicines. Most pharmacists probably feel the same way I do.

Good questions to ask your pharmacist when your child has a new medicine include:

- What is the name—both the trade name and the generic name—of the medicine?

- What strength is it (such as how many milligrams)?

- What is the medicine for? How does it work in the body?

- How many times a day do I give it? Does it matter what times of the day I give it (such as not close to bedtime, or at bedtime)?

- What should I do if I forget to give a dose of medicine to my child?

- Is this a medicine to give on a regular schedule or only when needed?

- Do I give the medicine by mouth (orally) or another way?

- Is a liquid form of the medicine available (for a young child)? If so, how does it taste? Can it be flavored?

- If the medicine is a tablet or capsule, can it be broken, crushed, or mixed with food to give to a young child?

- Where should I store this medicine: in the refrigerator or at room temperature?

- Should it be given with or without food, or is this not important?

- Are there any foods I should avoid giving my child because of this medicine?

- How long will the medicine have to be given: 7 to 10 days, 3 months, years?

- When will the medicine begin to help my child: immediately, in 1 to 2 weeks, or longer?

- How will I know if the medicine is helping my child? What should I look for?

- What are the most common side effects of the medicine? Are there any more serious but less common side effects? What can I do to lessen the risk of these side effects? What should I do if these side effects occur? Should I stop giving the medicine to my child?

- Is a generic form of the medicine available?

- Does this medicine have refills? If yes, how many?

- Is there anything special my child should not do, or be careful doing, when taking this medicine (such as driving, for an adolescent)?

- Does this medicine interact with or affect any of the other medicines my child is taking?

I have spoken with many parents who can't remember the names of the medicines their children take. To avoid this situation, it's a good idea to carry a list of your children's medicines in your wallet or purse. Write down the name of the medicine, its strength in milligrams (mgs) or grams (gms), and how many times each day it is given. This information may be especially useful if you change doctors or move to another area, because your child's medical records may take some time to obtain or transfer.

What questions about my child's medicine should I ask my child's doctor?

Before you leave your child's doctor's office, be sure that you have answers to several basic questions about any new medicines that were prescribed. Many of these questions are similar to those you should ask your pharmacist:

- What is the name—both the trade name and the generic name—of the medicine?

- What is the medicine for?

- How many times a day do I give it? Is this a medicine to give on a regular schedule, or only when needed?

- How and when will I know if the medicine is helping?

- How long should it be given? Only for a few days, or longer?

- What are the side effects of this medicine? What should I do if they occur? Should I call your office if any of these side effects occur?

- Is a generic form of this medicine available?

- Is this medicine expensive? Does my health insurance cover it? If not, are there other, similar medicines that my health insurance will cover better? (While this is a good question to ask, your doctor's nurse may be better able to answer this question than your doctor.)

- For younger children, is a liquid form of this medicine available? If so, how does it taste?

- Is this medicine given by mouth, or another way?

- Does this medicine interact with my child's other medicines?

- Does this medicine have refills?

Can Parents Use Expired Medicines in Some Circumstances?

I have a bottle of Motrin (ibuprofen) liquid that expired two weeks ago. Can I still use it?

Many parents wonder whether they can use medicine that has an expired date on it. Most medicines are not likely to be dangerous if used after their expiration date, but they can lose potency (strength), which means that they may not work as well. The manufacturer's expiration date is usually stamped in print on the medicine label or stamped on the bottom or side of the bottle or box. It may look like this: *EXP 10/12*. The date that the manufacturer places on the bottle or package is the latest date that the medicine should be used when it is stored and kept in appropriate conditions. How and where the medicine should be stored is described on the medicine bottle or box.

Medicine that is put into a bottle or vial at the pharmacy is usually given an expiration date of one year from the date that the prescription was filled. This expiration date is usually printed on the pharmacy label. Even if the original bottle of medicine at the pharmacy has an expiration date longer than one year, pharmacies put a one-year expiration date on the label because the medicine may not be stored in appropriate conditions in the patient's home.

Most medicines should be stored at room temperature in a dry, cool place. Unfortunately, many people keep their medicines in the bathroom, which is not a good place. Why is the bathroom, in the "medicine cabinet," not a good place? Bathrooms can have a lot of moisture in the air from use of the shower and bathtub. Moisture can degrade, or change, the chemicals in the medicine. It is better to keep your medicine in another room, such as a bedroom, and out of direct sunlight.

Some medicines should be stored in the refrigerator. Many liquid antibiotics are supposed to be stored in the refrigerator. Refrigerating liquid antibiotics often makes them taste better as well, which, as a parent, you already know is important! A few liquid antibiotics, however, should not be kept in the refrigerator because it may make them very thick and hard to pour from the bottle. Always ask at the pharmacy where you should store your child's medicine at home. If your child's medicine is supposed to be stored in the refrigerator and you accidentally leave it out overnight or during the day for a few hours, the medicine may still be safe to use. Call your pharmacy and ask.

So should you use that bottle of ibuprofen if it has a two-week-old expiration date? The best answer is to buy a new bottle and not use the older bottle. However, if it's late at night and your child has a fever, and an open pharmacy is not close by, and if you stored the ibuprofen in an appropriate place, it's reasonable to use the two-week-old bottle. Getting a newer bottle the next day would be a good idea.

What Do Mothers Need to Know about Taking Medications while Breast-feeding?

Breast-feeding and human milk are good for your baby in many ways. Breast-feeding provides good nutrition and protection from many types of infections (such as diarrhea, ear infections, and dangerous infections of the brain known as meningitis). It may also reduce the risk of SIDS (sudden infant death syndrome), and human milk may be able to help your baby's brain develop. Breast-feeding is also good for you as a mother, as it may decrease postpartum (after birth) bleeding and help you get back to your prepregnancy weight. For all these reasons, the American Academy of Pediatrics strongly supports breast-feeding for infants.

If you are taking medicine, even just a few tablets of an over-the-counter medicine, and you are breast-feeding your infant, you may have questions about how safe it is for your baby.

Is it possible that some of the medicine I am taking will get into my milk, and into my baby? Is it safe for my baby if I take this medicine?

Most medicines do get into breast milk, but in very small amounts, and for most medicines, such amounts are likely to be safe for your baby. Some medicines, however, should probably be avoided, if possible, when you breast-feed your baby. Fortunately, the medicines to avoid are few in number. There are not a lot of good scientific studies that can tell us how much of many of the available medicines get into breast milk.

If you are breast-feeding your infant, it is always a good idea to ask your doctor and pharmacist about specific medicines you are taking, or newly prescribed medicines, before you take them and breast-feed. You should ask about over-the-counter medicines as well. Factors that may affect how much of a medicine gets into breast milk and how much your infant may get include your infant's age, the volume of milk your infant eats, and the unique way your own body metabolizes (chemically changes) the medicine you take. How your infant metabolizes the medicine is also important.

Keep in mind these points while you are breast-feeding your infant and taking medicine:

1. Take your medicine at a time when you are not as likely to be breast-feeding your infant. For example, take your medicine just after you have breast-fed your infant or when you expect your infant to sleep for several hours. This allows the medicine to reach its highest concentration (amount) in your blood and milk when your infant will not be breast-feeding.

2. Use "short-acting" medicines when possible. Some medicine products are made to last longer, so they can be taken only once or twice per day. Many of these medicines are also available as short-acting products, which means that they often need to be taken three or more times per day. These short-acting products don't stay in your blood as long, which is preferred when you are breast-feeding.

3. Always closely watch your infant for any change in behavior if you are taking medicine and breast-feeding. For example, if your infant is sleeping much more, or less, since you started taking a medicine, it is possible that some of the medicine is getting into your milk and affecting your infant.

As I described above, many medicines are safe for you to use while you are breast-feeding your infant. When taking medicine—even medicines considered to be safe—follow the important points described above. Although it is safest not to take medicine while breast-feeding, there may be times when you need a medicine for your health. The following commonly used medicines are generally considered safe to use while breast-feeding (as long as you take an appropriate amount and not too much):

- acetaminophen (such as Tylenol) for headaches, pain, fever;
- ibuprofen (such as Motrin and Advil) for headaches, pain, fever;
- loratadine (such as Claritin) for allergies;
- dextromethorphan, a cough suppressant in many over-the-counter products (don't use liquid products that also contain alcohol); and
- many others (ask your doctor or pharmacist).

Some medicines may be more likely to have side effects in your infant if you take them and breast-feed. Fortunately, this list of medicines is short. Breast-feeding is probably best not done while a mother takes some of these medicines; with others on this list, it still may be possible for a mother to take them, if the infant is closely watched and monitored for medication side effects. (In other words, the benefit may be greater than the risk, as described in chapter 1.) These medicines include:

- medicines for cancer (it is usually best for a mother not to breast-feed if she needs a medicine for cancer);
- some medicines for seizure disorders;
- lithium carbonate for some psychiatric disorders (lithium carbonate can get into breast milk in a high amount, and it may cause side effects in an infant; however, it still may be possible for a breast-feeding mother to use lithium carbonate if the infant is closely monitored by a doctor);
- some medicines, such as some oral contraceptives (birth control pills), which may decrease the amount of milk a mother makes; and
- several others (ask your doctor or pharmacist).

Your doctor and pharmacist are your best sources of information about whether it is safe to use a specific medicine while you are breast-feeding your infant. They can refer to several books and other references about medicine use and breast-feeding to answer your questions. Many pharmacies have at least one of these books. Don't hesitate to ask us about this. Web sites for additional information about using medicine while breast-feeding include the www.healthychildren.org (American Academy of Pediatrics) and www.motherisk.org (Hospital for Sick Children at the University of Toronto). The Motherisk site can be especially helpful, and you may be able to call and speak with a counselor about specific questions you have about taking medicine and breast-feeding.

What Are the Essential Steps in Poison Prevention?

My 18-month-old daughter is walking well now, and she seems to want to put everything in her mouth. How can I prevent her from finding and taking too much medicine?

As infants become toddlers and learn to walk, they become very curious and can easily get into trouble and hurt themselves. Toddlers and young children like to put things in their mouths, and every parent probably has stories about what their children have stuck in their mouths. I recall when my son was young and we were in the backyard on a nice summer day. When I picked him up, he appeared to have something in his mouth. I looked inside and saw he was sucking on a small rock like it was a piece of candy. Not too long after that, I was with him on the sidewalk next to our house when he reached down to pick something up from the grass and was about to put it into his mouth. I grabbed his hand—he had a piece of dog poop!

So if infants and young children will put nearly anything into their mouths, they may also put medicine into their mouths. Even just a small amount of some medicines can be deadly to a young child. Some medicines that have very few side effects and are very safe to use in infants and children for medical reasons can be deadly if too large an amount is taken (this is called a toxic dose). A good example is acetaminophen (such as Tylenol). Acetaminophen is a very commonly used medicine in children, and when it is given in an appropriate amount to treat fever or pain, it is safe and has few side effects. However, too much acetaminophen (a toxic dose) may cause severe damage to the liver, which can be deadly. Less than one bottle (3.4 ounces) of children's acetaminophen liquid suspension contains enough acetaminophen to be potentially deadly to a 30-pound, 2-year-old child if he or she were to drink most of the bottle. Childhood poisonings are completely avoidable, and you can prevent your child from becoming accidentally poisoned with medicine.

It can take only a few minutes for your child to get hold of some medicine and take too much. This often happens when you or other adults are distracted or not paying attention to what children are doing. What can you do as a parent to reduce the risk of medicine poisoning in your children? You can help to protect your children if you:

- Keep ALL your medicines in a safe place: up high and away from the reach of children, and not easily found.
- Keep ALL medicines in their original containers with the label describing the bottle contents, and keep child-resistant tops closed tightly.
- Put ALL medicines safely away once you are finished using them. Don't leave them around to "use later."
- Assume that ALL medicines can be dangerous to your children and store them safely. Even medicines that are "safe" when used correctly, such as acetaminophen or iron or vitamins, can be deadly to young children if they take too much.
- Use cabinet safety locks to keep children out of floor-level and waist-level cabinets in your home.
- Store other potentially dangerous substances in your home safely. This includes household cleaners, insect repellents, and car windshield wiper fluids.

Don't forget about other homes where your children can find medicines. Perhaps the best example is grandma and grandpa's home. Many grandmas and grandpas take several medicines for their health, and some of these medicines can be especially dangerous to young children. Adults' medicines often have easy-open tops on the medicine bottles, and the medicine bottles are often kept in the kitchen or other rooms in the home. If you are going to grandma and grandpa's home, ask them to put their medicines away in a safe place before you arrive with your children.

One of the most important points to remember about childhood poisoning is the phone number to call if your child has found some medicine and taken it. The phone number of all the national poison control centers is the best number to call: 1-800-222-1222. If your child is not breathing or is unconscious, call 911.

How Should Parents Give Children Medicine Orally, in the Nose, in the Ear, and in the Eye?

Giving medicine to an infant or child can be quite a challenge. You may have a safe and effective medicine to give your child, but if he or she will not take it, the medicine will not help. Chapter 2 described some reliable ways to give medicine to a child. Here I provide specific instructions for giving medicine to your child by mouth, in the nose, in the ear, and in the eye.

General Tips on Giving Medicine (see chapter 2 for more information)

1. Use an appropriate measuring device for giving liquid oral medicine, such as an oral dosing syringe or an infant measuring dropper.
2. For infants, have another adult hold the infant, including his or her arms. For older infants or young children, place them in an infant car seat or high chair used for eating.
3. Wash your hands before giving medicine to your child.
4. If your child resists, try distracting her. Use a favorite television show or video, or have another adult or older child blow bubbles or do something else to distract your child.

HOW TO GIVE LIQUID MEDICINE ORALLY

For infants and young children, I believe that it's best to use an infant medicine dropper or an oral dosing syringe. If the medicine product has a dropper or dosing syringe in the box package, use it. Droppers and oral syringes are better to use, as they are less likely to spill the medicine (as compared to a dosing spoon). You may have to shake the liquid medicine bottle first (see the label or package).

1. Place the dropper or oral syringe into your child's mouth. Slowly push or squirt the liquid medicine into the *side* of your child's mouth. Do not

quickly squirt the liquid medicine into the back of your child's mouth, as he or she may choke. Young children may want to help by holding the oral syringe or by sucking the medicine out of the oral syringe.

2. If for some reason your child does not seem to be swallowing the medicine, you can try gently holding his or her cheeks together and then lightly stroking under the chin.

3. When done, rinse the dropper or oral syringe with water. Don't let your child play with any device, as he or she could potentially choke on it. Store it in a safe place.

HOW TO GIVE MEDICINE IN THE NOSE
Nose liquid drops (you may have to shake the bottle first, if the label says so):

1. It's best to clear your child's nose first. For an infant, use a bulb syringe and suck out the mucus. For an older child, have him or her blow the nose with a tissue.

2. If the medicine is stored in the refrigerator, warm it up first by holding the bottle and rolling it in your hands for a few minutes.

3. For an infant, hold your child as he or she is lying down with the head tilted back a little bit. For an older child, have him or her lie down and tilt the head back a little bit as well. A pillow may help for an older child (place the pillow under the child's upper back, so the head can tilt over the pillow).

4. With the medicine in the dropper, place the dropper just slightly into the nostril. Try not to touch the nostril with the dropper, although this may be difficult. Place the medicine drops into the nostril(s).

5. Keep your infant or child lying down for 1 or 2 minutes after putting the drops in. An older child may tell you that he or she can taste the medicine in the throat. This is normal. If he or she feels like spitting because of the taste, this is not a problem and you can allow the child to spit.

HOW TO GIVE MEDICINE IN THE EAR
Ear liquid drops (you may have to shake the bottle first, if the label says so):

1. If the medicine is stored in the refrigerator, warm it up first by holding the bottle and rolling it in your hands for a few minutes.

2. Place your child on his or her side, with the ear facing up.

3. For younger children (younger than 3 years), pull the ear lobe back and down. For older children (3 years and older), pull the upper ear lobe back and up.

4. Place the medicine from the dropper into the ear canal. Try not to touch the ear with the dropper.

5. Keep your child lying in this position for about 2 minutes. You can place a cotton plug into the ear to help keep the medicine in place if your child will not stay still.

HOW TO GIVE MEDICINE IN THE EYE
Eye liquid drops and ointment (you may have to shake the bottle of liquid first, if the label says so):

1. If the medicine is stored in the refrigerator, warm it up first by holding the bottle and rolling it in your hands for a few minutes.

2. Lie your younger child down. Using a warm, moist washcloth or cotton, gently wipe and clean the eyes. An older child can stand up for this part.

3. Gently pull the lower eyelid down until you see a small pouch. Without touching the medicine dropper to the eye, place the liquid drop into this pouch. If the directions are for more than one drop per eye, wait about 1 minute before putting in the next drop.

4. An older child can stand and tilt the head back. Ask your child to look straight up and gently pull the lower eyelid down until you see a small pouch. Without touching the medicine dropper to the eye, place the liquid drop into this pouch. If the directions are for more than one drop per eye, wait about 1 minute before putting in the next drop.

5. Try to keep your younger child lying down for a few minutes after putting the eye drops in or have your older child close the eyes for about 1 minute.

6. For eye ointments, use the same directions as above. Pull down the lower eyelid until you see a pouch, and then place a line of the ointment medicine into the length of this pouch. Try not to touch the tip of the ointment tube to the eye. Gently move or jiggle the ointment tube as you are nearly done, so the ointment will drop off the end of the tube. Try to keep your child lying down for a few minutes after putting in the ointment, or have your older child close the eyes for about 1 minute.

You can easily find this information about how to give medicines to children on several Web sites. Not all of the information on these sites may be accurate, however. I recommend using the Web sites of the American Academy of Pediatrics (www.aap.org and www.healthychildren.org) or the Pediatric Pharmacy Advocacy Group (www.kidsmeds.info). The Pediatric Pharmacy Advocacy Group is a professional organization of pediatric pharmacists, of which I am a member.

Best of luck, and happy parenting to all parents out there!

REFERENCES

CHAPTER 1. Should I Give Medicine to My Child?

G. L. Kearns, "Developmental pharmacology: Drug disposition, action, and therapy in infants and children," *New England Journal of Medicine,* September 2003.

E. A. Bell and D. E. Tunkel, "Over-the-counter cough and cold medications in children: Are they helpful?" *Otolaryngology and Head and Neck Surgery,* May 2010.

CHAPTER 2. How Should I Give Medicine to My Child?

E. A. Bell, "Tastes of liquid medications: Pediatric implications," *Journal of Pediatric Pharmacology and Therapeutics,* January 1999.

D. M. Kraus, "Effectiveness and infant acceptance of the Rx medibottle versus the oral syringe," *Pharmacotherapy,* April 2001.

W. T. Zempsky, "Pharmacologic approaches for reducing venous access pain in children," *Pediatrics,* November 2008.

CHAPTER 3. How Do I Use Medicines for Fever?

M. Crocetti, "Fever phobia revisited: Have parental misconceptions about fever changed in 20 years?" *Pediatrics,* June 2001.

E. M. Sarrell, "Antipyretic treatment in young children with fever," *Archives of Pediatrics and Adolescent Medicine,* February 2006.

L. C. Kramer, "Alternating antipyretics: Antipyretic efficacy of acetaminophen versus acetaminophen alternated with ibuprofen in children," *Clinical Pediatrics,* November 2008.

S. M. Lesko, "An assessment of the safety of pediatric ibuprofen," *Journal of the American Medical Association,* March 1995.

M. D. S. Erlewyn-Lajeunesse, "Randomized controlled trial of combined paracetamol and ibuprofen for fever," *Archives of Diseases of Childhood*, May 2006.

American Academy of Pediatrics, "Clinical report: Fever and antipyretic use in children," *Pediatrics*, March 2011.

CHAPTER 4. How Do I Use Medicines for Infection?

P. J. Louhiala, "Form of day care and respiratory infections among Finnish children," *American Journal of Public Health*, August 1995.

A. E. Aiello, "Consumer antibacterial soaps: Effective or just risky?" *Clinical Infectious Diseases*, Supplement 2, 2007.

G. M. Lee, "Illness transmission in the home: A possible role for alcohol-based hand gels," *Pediatrics*, April 2005.

E. M. Sarrell, "Efficacy of naturopathic extracts in the management of ear pain associated with acute otitis media," *Archives of Pediatrics and Adolescent Medicine*, July 2001.

E. A. Bell, "Over-the-counter cough and cold medications in children: Are they helpful?" *Otolaryngology and Head and Neck Surgery*, May 2010.

I. A. Paul, "Effect of honey, dextromethorphan, and no treatment on nocturnal cough and sleep quality for coughing children and their parents," *Archives of Pediatrics and Adolescent Medicine*, December 2007.

H. S. Yin, "Evaluation of consistency in dosing directions and measuring devices for pediatric nonprescription liquid medications," *Journal of the American Medical Association*, December 2010.

I. A. Paul, "Vapor rub, petrolatum, and no treatment for children with nocturnal cough and cold symptoms," *Pediatrics*, December 2010.

American Academy of Pediatrics, "Clinical report: Probiotics and prebiotics in pediatrics," *Pediatrics*, December 2010.

P. A. Tahtinen, "A placebo-controlled trial of antimicrobial treatment for acute otitis media," *New England Journal of Medicine*, January 2011.

A. Hoberman, "Treatment of acute otitis media in children under 2 years of age," *New England Journal of Medicine*, January 2011.

CHAPTER 5. Are Vaccines Dangerous? Will They Protect My Child?

K. M. Madsen, "A population-based study of measles, mumps, and rubella vaccination and autism," *New England Journal of Medicine*, November 2002.

P. J. Smith, "Parental delays, refusals for vaccines up in survey," *Infectious Diseases in Children*, May 2010.

K. Wilson, "Association of autistic spectrum disorder and the measles, mumps, and rubella vaccine: A systemic review of current epidemiological evidence," *Archives of Pediatrics and Adolescent Medicine*, April 2003.

G. L. Freed, "Parental vaccine safety concerns in 2009," *Pediatrics*, April 2010.

D. Mrozek-Budzyn, "Lack of association between measles-mumps-rubella vaccination and autism in children," *Pediatric Infectious Disease Journal*, May 2010.

CHAPTER 6. How Do I Use Medicines for Common Illnesses?

C. K. King, "Managing acute gastroenteritis among children, oral rehydration, maintenance, and nutritional therapy," *Morbidity and Mortality Weekly Report*, November 2003.

American Academy of Pediatrics, "Clinical report: Head lice," *Pediatrics*, August 2010.

S. Pedersen, "Clinical safety of inhaled corticosteroids for asthma," *Drug Safety*, July 2006.

L. Agertoft, "Effect of long-term treatment with inhaled budesonide on adult height in children with asthma," *New England Journal of Medicine*, October 2000.

A. M. W. Floet, "Attention-deficit hyperactivity disorder," *Pediatrics in Review*, February 2010.

National Heart, Lung, and Blood Institute, "Guidelines for the diagnosis and management of asthma," *National Institutes of Health*, July 2007.

INDEX